NO
IF'S, AND'S OR
BUTTS

NO
IF'S, AND'S OR
BUTTS

The Smoker's Guide to
QUITTING

Harlan M. Krumholz, MD
Robert H. Phillips, PhD

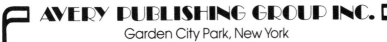

AVERY PUBLISHING GROUP INC.

Garden City Park, New York

The medical information presented in his book is not intended as a substitute for consulting your physician. All matters regarding your physical health should be supervised by a health-care professional. Because the information in this field is constantly expanding and changing, the publisher and authors urge you to stay abreast of new techniques and products as they become available.

Cover design: The Morris-Lee Group
Editor: Liza Burby
Typesetter: Bonnie Freid

Library of Congress Cataloging-in-Publication Data

Krumholz, Harlan M.
    No if's, and's, or butts : the smoker's guide to quitting /
Harlan M. Krumholz, Robert H. Phillips.
      p. cm.
    Includes index.
    ISBN 0-89529-534-2
    1. Cigarette smokers—Rehabilitation. 2. Tobacco
habit—Treatment.   I. Phillips, Robert H., 1948– .   II. Title.
HV5740.K78 1993
613.85—dc20   92-39845
                                   CIP

Printed in the United States of America

10 9 8 7 6 5 4 3 2 1

Contents

To those who have the courage to try
and the wisdom to prepare.

Acknowledgments

This book would not have been possible without the contribution of many people. I am grateful to my father, Richard A. Krumholz, M.D., who envisioned this book as a helping hand to smokers who want to quit. It was the love and support of my wife, Leslie, and my children, Samuel, Rebecca, and Sarah, that allowed me to complete the project. Others who provided valuable assistance and support include Susan Klein, Steve Mufson, Gloria Haffer, Lois Rosenthal, Carol Balnicki, Dace Jansons, Larry Barbaras, Ken Rogers, Robert Glickman, M.D., Richard Pasternak, M.D., Jane Weeks, M.D., Martha Wilson, Elise Phillips, Susan Ridker, Paul Ridker, M.D., Lynne Krumholz, Julie Krumholz, Sylvia Heyman, and Ken and Elaine Roberts. Finally, I am indebted to our publisher, Rudy Shur, who believed in the importance of this book from the beginning and helped to bring it to completion.

Harlan M. Krumholz, M.D.

This book is lovingly dedicated to the special people in my life: my wife; my three sons; my parents, sister, and grandparents; my other relatives and in-laws; and my friends, all of whom I'd like to see live life in a healthy, smoke-free environment. I am grateful for the support and assistance of my Center for Coping staff, especially Ann Dominger, Michelle Walsh, Helena LaValley, and Melissa Sheinwold, in the processing, editing, and preparation necessary for the completion of this book.

Robert H. Phillips, Ph.D.

Preface

Preparation is the important foundation for success in all endeavors. Quitting smoking, one of the greatest challenges you can undertake, requires no less. We started this book because of our belief that many smokers fail in their attempts to quit their habit because they are not adequately prepared to succeed.

No If's, And's, or Butts was written to provide you with the opportunity to learn about smoking cessation. Many smokers have not had this chance. As a result, some have been lured by unproven products that make fantastic claims and prey on the trust of smokers, and others have missed the opportunity to benefit from some truly helpful programs, techniques, and strategies.

Let us help you to take advantage of the best medical and scientific information on how to quit. Much of this valuable information does not make it to the public—to those smokers who could use it most. Even many physicians do not know as much as they should about how to help their patients quit smoking. Much has been learned about methods to quit smoking in the more than twenty-five years since the release of the first *Surgeon General's Report on the Health Consequences of Smoking*. Research careers have been devoted to evaluating various methods and determining what works and what does not. Take advantage of this knowledge. Invest some time with this book and develop your personalized quit-smoking program, based on solid medical and scientific information.

Although this book cannot quit smoking for you, it can help you to help yourself. While the ultimate responsibility for success rests with you, we can prepare you to succeed by helping you combine your will power with powerful information about quitting. Will power and knowledge are a very potent combination.

There is hope for every smoker. Millions of people have quit. You can join them. This is the first step.

Introduction

Do you like to smoke but want to (or feel you should) quit? Are you excited about stopping, or are you afraid you won't be able to? Regardless, this book is the place to start! As a smoker who would like to give up cigarettes, you are not alone. Surveys suggest that most smokers would like to be free from cigarettes and that many of them have tried unsuccessfully to quit many times.

Millions of Americans smoke. Some of them have never tried to stop; many others have been unable to stop. However, it is not impossible to quit! Over 30 million Americans *have* succeeded in giving up cigarettes! If you would like to stop, either now or eventually, the information presented in this book should be of tremendous benefit.

HOW STRONG IS YOUR MOTIVATION?

Do you really want to stop? Imagine this scenario: You have found a magic pill. If you take it, you would wake up tomorrow morning as a nonsmoker—and you wouldn't miss it. Would you take the pill? If, like most people, you would be thrilled to, then you really do want to stop smoking. But maybe you're afraid. Maybe you don't have confidence in yourself. Maybe you're concerned about all the possible side effects. Don't let that stop you. Whatever your concerns are, with the right preparation, you can succeed!

THE IMPORTANCE OF PLANNING

How many important goals have you tried to achieve without preparation? Probably very few, if any. So doesn't it make sense, for this life-extending goal, to combine your commitment to quit with a practical plan of action? If you want to learn about all of the current popular methods of smoking cessation, and if you want to develop a strategy that fits your needs and helps you to succeed in your quest to quit, then this book is for you.

Unfortunately, too many people try to quit smoking without a plan. They don't do their homework, nor do they take advantage of the thousands of scientific studies about smoking and smoking cessation. They don't take time to learn which techniques have the potential to help them and which ones will waste their time. Many smokers try to quit cold turkey. They feel that their success rests solely on their will power.

Smokers are often discouraged after a failed attempt to quit and many berate themselves for being a "loser." If you have felt this, then you are not alone. If, however, you have tried to quit without learning all you can about smoking-cessation techniques, then you started at a disadvantage. There are no magic methods, but there are plenty of good ones available. Wouldn't it help to know which methods to consider and which methods to avoid?

Quitting is far from a simple activity. You certainly know that, especially if you're reading this book. But knowledge about cigarette cessation is a powerful tool. No, this knowledge doesn't guarantee your success. But it does allow you to have an edge in this very important life challenge. There are significant differences between the methods available. Even if you're planning to quit on your own, there are simple key techniques you can use to improve your chances of success.

WHAT THIS BOOK CAN AND CANNOT DO FOR YOU

Unfortunately, this book cannot provide you with some secret formula for success. No one has discovered the difference between the smokers who fail in their attempt to quit and those who succeed. Furthermore, no program or technique has emerged as the single best way to quit. If there were one best way, you would certainly have heard about it. In fact, you should be wary of anyone who makes seemingly unbelievable claims about a program.

It is our strong belief that preparation is one of your greatest allies in your attempt to quit. What this book can do for you is to help you prepare to succeed by teaching you about smoking and smoking-cessation strategies and helping you design a personalized program. It can provide you with the latest up-to-date information about the programs, techniques, and devices that can make your attempt to stop smoking a successful one. This book is written for the millions of smokers who would like to quit and want to maximize their chances of success.

No If's, And's, or Butts is divided into three parts. The first part will set the stage for your life-extending decision to stop smoking. You'll learn about the phases of smoking cessation as well as the reasons for its difficulty. You can probably cite the reasons already, but you'll learn much more about yourself that will help you immeasurably.

A review of all the latest smoking-cessation techniques, programs, and devices will be found in the second part of the book. You'll become aware of all the effective (and not-so-effective) techniques that are currently available. This information will, hopefully, help you become an educated consumer who can decide which methods are beneficial and which are not.

Finally, the third part of the book will help you put your own unique smoking-cessation program into effect. You'll learn how to quit and, even more importantly, how to remain a nonsmoker!

Use this book both as a source of information and for support. Use it as a guide to success. First read through the book in its entirety. Then go back and reread the sections that are most applicable to you. Take notes, and write your plans and goals in the margins. Make the book work for you.

Part I
Preparing to Quit

CHAPTER 1

The Stages of Quitting

Congratulations! You've decided to quit smoking. Let's make this desire a reality! We know if it were easy to stop smoking, then you wouldn't need this book. But it is *not* easy. Many ex-smokers have claimed that stopping was one of the hardest things they ever had to do! So let's do it right. Let's accomplish this goal once and for all.

QUITTING IS A PROCESS

Recognize that quitting is not so much an event as it is a process. In other words, smoking cessation is not something that "takes place" and then is over. "Sure," you might say, "one minute you have a cigarette and the next minute you don't." But the process of stopping—and then, more importantly, remaining a nonsmoker—is continuous. To be successful, you will have to consciously work on this process for a long, long time. This is not meant to scare you; rather, it's meant to prepare you. If you really and truly want to quit smoking, you need to know exactly what you are facing. You need to prepare yourself as best you can for any obstacle you may encounter along the way. You can gain from your experience and the experiences of others as you begin to quit smoking.

HOW TO BEGIN

Start by looking at where you are. Why are you reading this book? Was it your choice to buy it? Or was it given to you by someone who has been pressuring you to quit? When would you like to be a nonsmoker? Are you thinking of quitting within the next six months? Would you like to quit during the next thirty days? Have you tried to quit before? What is the longest period that you have stayed away from cigarettes? These important questions provide some insight into your relationship with cigarettes. (Yes, breaking up is hard to do!)

THE FOUR STAGES OF QUITTING

The process of smoking cessation has been researched extensively. From time to time, we will refer to some of these studies. We are not trying to bore you. We are trying to present you with the latest conclusions drawn by experts who are (almost) as interested in your being successful at quitting as you are.

The process of giving up smoking can best be outlined as four stages: pre-contemplation, contemplation, action, and maintenance. Many smokers go through these stages a number of times. Your ultimate goal is to go through the four stages and successfully remain in the maintenance stage.

Let's discuss these four stages in more detail.

First Stage: Pre-Contemplation

Remember when you were not really thinking about quitting? You may even have been annoyed by suggestions that you should quit. When you were feeling like this, you were actually in the first stage. At this point, you did not have any conscious plans to quit within the next six months. In fact, in this stage, you may have been actively resistant to quitting. Pleas from your family and friends went unheeded and may have made you hostile. Doctors may have advised you to stop, but this advice was rejected or sidestepped. Information about the harms of smoking was avoided or ignored. The pre-contemplation stage could also be appropriately called the avoidance or denial stage.

Second Stage: Contemplation

The second stage is called contemplation. In this stage, you become willing to contemplate, or consider, the idea of smoking cessation. You have become concerned about your health and are worried about the unhealthy side effects of smoking. But to legitimately be in this stage, you must seriously be considering quitting within the next six months.

The contemplation stage is a critically important time. It is now that you decide whether to go on to the next stage of quitting or to continue smoking, in some cases even returning to the pre-contemplation stage. Once the decision is made, many smokers forge ahead to attempt quitting because they do not want to lose their momentum. Although this may work for a few smokers, most benefit from pausing in the contemplation stage. Why? Because you really need to prepare yourself for success. If your momentum is so fleeting that you believe you must move ahead or lose your nerve, then you are probably not really ready to quit. Your success is likely to be short-lived.

Why is it so important to pause in the contemplation stage? No one would attempt a marathon and expect to finish unless he or she had adequately prepared. The challenge of quitting smoking is no different. Now is the time to learn everything you can about quitting cigarettes in order to maximize your chances of success.

Third Stage: Action

This is the stage during which you act on your decision to quit. What does this mean? During the action stage, you start the actual behavioral process of quitting, or at least you constructively prepare for it. In this stage, you set a specific date to quit and select the specific smoking-cessation method. All your preparation has been completed and you know how, when, and what you are going to do. This is the critical transitional stage, when you change from a smoker to an ex-smoker.

Fourth Stage: Maintenance

You've taken the "plunge." You've stopped smoking. But you want to remain an ex-smoker, right? That is why the fourth stage, called maintenance, is the most important one. During this stage, you want to maintain your status as an ex-smoker and avoid a relapse into the old familiar behavior of smoking.

This is also the time when you must fend off the cravings, urges, and temptations, and maintain your abstinence.

If you are completely successful, the maintenance stage is the last one. Your ultimate goal is to stay in this stage for the rest of your life and never smoke again. That is why most people feel that this is the most difficult stage.

WHAT STAGE ARE YOU IN?

If you are reading this book, you're probably in the contemplation stage. You're considering stopping. True, you may have tried before, but if so, you're considering *again!*

Many people have mixed feelings at this point. They ask themselves, "Should I or shouldn't I? Do I really want to stop or would I rather continue smoking?" This confusion probably won't disappear until after you have successfully stopped. Some ex-smokers continue to have mixed feelings. But if you know that stopping is the right choice, don't let your mixed feelings interfere with your success at quitting.

So what is your first goal? You want to move from contemplation to action—from thinking about quitting to actively doing something about it! The rest of this book will help you to accomplish this by teaching you how to overcome obstacles to action and by giving you suggestions both to motivate you and to improve your chances of success. It will help you to determine what kind of smoking-cessation action will be best for you.

FROM CONTEMPLATION TO ACTION

If you want to quit smoking, the first question to ask yourself is, *"Am I ready?"* This question is the first step. Why? Because any effort is wasted unless you feel ready to make this important change in your life.

To some degree, you are ready. How do we know? Well, you are reading this book, aren't you? You are at least thinking about quitting. Take a moment and give yourself some credit. You have already made an important change. Some smokers never even make it this far! To open your mind to the possibility that you can free yourself from cigarettes is your first victory. (If you have tried before and failed, forget about it. Scientific studies have shown that the number of previous failed attempts says nothing about your ability to quit now. Plus, this time you are going to be prepared to succeed. So, instead of dwelling on past failures, start anew immediately!)

While it's great that you're contemplating "the big move" now, don't rest on the success of making it this far. Keep moving. Your next goal is to decide to act and to begin actively preparing to quit. This objective, however, is often not easily achieved. Many smokers come to the brink of deciding to quit only to retreat from the idea. Has this happened to you? It's like pausing on the edge of an ice-cold swimming pool on a hot day. You know you will feel good when you are finally in and have adjusted to the temperature, but you are afraid of that initial icy plunge!

What should you do if you are having trouble moving from contemplation to action? First, don't be discouraged. It is normal to be uncertain. Give your decision some thought. Learn more about smoking and why you smoke. (Read the rest of Part I of this book.) Focus your attention on the reasons to quit. If, after all your contemplation, you are not yet ready to quit, take a break, relax, regroup, and decide if you want to prepare again later. You can succeed and we can help you, but in your heart you must be ready to try.

TIME TO MOVE ON

Now it's time to move on to prepare for success. Remember the main goals of smoking cessation: You want to leave behind a habit that is both physically and emotionally harmful to you. You want to replace it with newer, more appropriate ways of enjoying life and for dealing with its difficult aspects. And you want to be more in control of your life, not enslaved to an addiction that has trapped you in the past. Now it's time to go after those goals. Good luck!

CHAPTER 2

Why Is It So Difficult to Quit?

Almost everyone who smokes finds it difficult to quit. Why? Because for millions of people, smoking is an ingrained behavior, a habit. Before we explain some of the reasons why, let's briefly discuss where smoking originated.

A BRIEF HISTORY OF TOBACCO

Tobacco was used by early cultures in the Western Hemisphere. They discovered ways to burn dried tobacco leaves and to inhale the smoke through a hollow reed. During intense religious ceremonies, a stuporous state resulted when a person either chewed the leaves or inhaled the smoke. People respected this ability of tobacco to alter moods, and the use of tobacco was restricted to sacred and religious ceremonies.

Europeans were introduced to inhaling tobacco smoke when they landed in the New World. It is said that the natives of the West Indies offered dried tobacco leaves to Christopher Columbus as a gift when he arrived in 1492. Initially, Europeans used tobacco for medicinal purposes. It is interesting to note that for many years, tobacco was believed to cure many ailments—including cancer!

The tobacco originally used by Native Americans was very harsh. The recreational use of tobacco by Europeans spread with the development of methods of growing and treating tobacco that resulted in a more pleasant smoke. For these advantages, we can thank John Rolfe (who married Pocahontas) and Sir Walter Raleigh.

Despite the popularity of smoking, its acceptance has never been universal. Even before the dangers of smoking were known with certainty, King James I of England was a vehement critic. In 1604, he called tobacco a "filthy weed" and described smoking as "loathsome to the eye, hateful to the nose, harmful to the brain, and dangerous to the lungs." His differences with Sir Walter Raleigh led to the abrupt end of Raleigh's smoking habit. Raleigh was beheaded!

Over the years, nevertheless, people have found many ways to use tobacco. It has been placed in the body through the nose (snuff), through the mouth (chewing tobacco), and through the lungs (smoke). Each method enjoyed its period of popularity. In the nineteenth century, most people who used tobacco preferred to chew it. In the twentieth century, smoking tobacco was more widespread. Mass production was perfected, and many companies made large profits from the smoking industry. The use of cigars, popular because they could be smoked as well as chewed, peaked in 1920 when 8 billion were sold. In the last fifty years, cigarettes have emerged as the most popular way to use tobacco.

SMOKING IN AMERICA

Cigarette smoking became an important part of American culture in the early part of the twentieth century. For a long time, the government participated in endorsing cigarettes. During World War II, the government distributed cigarettes as a gift to servicemen. Even President Franklin D. Roosevelt was famous for his smoking. He was often seen with his cigarette holder hanging out of the side of his mouth.

For centuries, only men were entitled to smoke cigarettes. As society gradually acknowledged the rights of women, the tobacco industry seized on a large untapped market. Marketing campaigns targeted women, who then also became frequent inhalers of tobacco smoke.

Business grew to meet the increased demand for cigarettes. Efficient machines replaced hand rollers. Fortunes were made, and tobacco became one of the country's most important cash crops. By the late 1960s, over half of the population smoked cigarettes and an average of over 4,000 cigarettes was sold annually for each adult in the United States! In 1983, cigarette sales in this country exceeded $630 billion.

THE REASONS PEOPLE SMOKE

There are many different reasons why people smoke. Each person gets his or her own unique satisfaction from it.

You know how difficult it can be to break a habit. With smoking, you are not only psychologically addicted, but you're also physiologically addicted, which compounds the problem. Your body as well as your mind has become dependent on nicotine. Almost all smokers develop this dependence. In fact, smokers of cigarettes without nicotine find smoking boring and distasteful, and quickly seek cigarettes with nicotine.

The challenge of quitting is even greater because of the billions of dollars spent on cigarette advertising. To quit, you must fight not only your dependence on nicotine but the subtle, yet persistent, messages from the tobacco industry. Cigarette companies don't want you to quit. You are up against tremendous advertising campaigns designed to keep you smoking their brands.

To give yourself the best chance of success, you should understand as much as possible about the power of cigarettes. Knowledge of your opponent is important for victory. This is a key ingredient to developing a strategy for success.

Smoking Addiction: Internal Influences

Smoking provides many types of sensory stimulation. These include the taste and smell of the cigarette as well as the slightly irritating stimulation of the nose and throat that can be perceived as pleasurable if it is associated with nicotine. In addition, there is stimulation from a tactile sensation, both in the hands and in the mouth.

Smokers all have a strong bond to cigarettes. This bond, however, is more than affection for a simple habit. Cigarette smoking is an addiction. Yes, it's true. Being addicted is one of the main reasons it is so difficult to quit. Recognizing that smoking is an addiction is the first step toward freedom from smoking.

Smoking hasn't always been seen as an addiction. For centuries, cigarette smoking was considered little more than a persistent but innocuous habit. Few people considered it a form of drug dependence. The idea that smoking could addict a person in a manner similar to morphine, cocaine, or alcohol was ridiculed.

Over the past twenty years, however, the more modern view of cigarettes has evolved. Currently, most experts consider cigarette smoking more of an addiction than a habit. In fact, national and international organizations, including the World Health Organization, the Royal College of Physicians, the American Psychiatric Association, and the United States Department of Health and Human Services, have stated that cigarette smoking is an addiction.

The 1988 *Surgeon General's Report* entitled "The Health Consequences of Smoking" was devoted to the subject of smoking and nicotine addiction. This 600-page report drew on the expertise of over 500 scientists and cited more than 2,500 articles. What did it conclude? Primarily that cigarettes and other forms of tobacco are addictive and that nicotine is the drug in tobacco that causes addiction.

Why is cigarette smoking considered an addiction?

To answer this question, let's consider exactly what an addiction is. Addictions involve the compulsive use of substances that affect your mood. The more you use an addictive substance, the more you want to continue using it, and the more physically dependent on it you become. You continue to use the substance despite its known harmful effects. Quitting the use of the substance becomes extremely difficult. If you quit, you frequently suffer relapses. It's important to understand that this description applies to cocaine, heroin, alcohol—and cigarettes.

You may not want to think about smoking this way. In comparison to heroin and cocaine, you might say, smoking seems relatively mild! That's true. Cigarettes do not cause the powerful chemical "high" of other psychoactive drugs. They do not negatively affect your ability to work or drive a car. Yet, there is no doubt that cigarettes produce a deep dependence. This dependence can only be called an addiction.

The distinction between a habit and an addiction is important. A habit implies an innocuous though persistent and sometimes bothersome activity that you can control. With an addiction, however, you find it extremely difficult to stop using a substance, even if you'd like to.

Think for a moment about how powerful addictive substances can be. What is it that drives an alcoholic to drink, even at the cost of his or her marriage, work, health, and self-esteem? What is it that compels a successful executive to risk his position, livelihood, and freedom for a line of cocaine? What is it that motivates a previously honest person to steal in order to pay for an expensive heroin habit? And, what is it that drives a sensible, intelligent person who would otherwise avoid risky situations to smoke cigarettes despite the well-publicized health dangers? These are the mysteries of addiction.

How does tobacco cause addiction?

Smoking, at its most basic level, is the repetitive exposure of the body to nicotine. Each puff gives you a small dose of nicotine, along with hundreds of other harmful chemicals. Smoking products that do not contain nicotine have never really been successfully marketed since smokers tend to shun them.

Smokers seem to need nicotine. Studies have shown that smokers will modify their behavior to maintain their intake of nicotine. If they are given cigarettes with a low nicotine yield, they will inhale more deeply, take more puffs, and smoke more cigarettes. Some smokers even discover that they can increase their exposure to nicotine by covering the holes in the filter and preventing the cigarette smoke from mixing with air. If smokers are given short cigarettes, they will smoke more of them. If they are treated with a medicine that causes their bodies to get rid of nicotine more rapidly, they will increase the number of cigarettes they smoke. If they are deprived of nicotine, they will crave it.

Smokers often fall into a rut called the addictive triad. For smokers, the components of this triad are developing the nicotine addiction, becoming dependent on it, and experiencing withdrawal symptoms when trying to stop.

What is nicotine?

Nicotine is a chemical substance found in tobacco leaves. It was named after Jean Nicot, a French statesman who used an extract of tobacco to treat a stomach ailment that Catherine de Medici, the queen of France, had in the 1560s.

When tobacco is burned, nicotine is carried on tar droplets in the tobacco smoke. It then goes to the lungs, where it is absorbed into the bloodstream. Alternatively, tobacco is sometimes placed in the mouth (chewing tobacco) or nose (snuff). In these ways, nicotine can be absorbed into the body without smoking. In each of these methods, nicotine reaches the brain and affects the mood. Most importantly, it eventually leads to a craving for more.

What are the immediate effects of nicotine?

In small doses, nicotine can act as a stimulant. This may make it seem like it is increasing your behavioral efficiency. In fact, nicotine increases the output of adrenaline, thereby increasing blood pressure and heart rate. The drug also affects the rate of body metabolism, temperature regulation, muscle relaxation, and the secretion of certain hormones. With continual smoking, nicotine quickly accumulates and remains in the body for over six hours.

What is so special about the role of cigarettes?

If you were challenged to develop a method that would deliver a dose of nicotine to the brain almost instantaneously, you could do no better than to invent smoking. Nicotine from a cigarette puff reaches your brain even faster than it would if it were injected into a vein using a syringe! Furthermore, over 90 percent of the nicotine inhaled in each puff enters the bloodstream, so cigarette smoking delivers nicotine not only quickly but also efficiently.

Cigarettes have another strength as a nicotine delivery system. They enable you to control exactly how much you take in. You can regulate both how deeply you inhale with each puff and how many puffs you take.

How do you know you are physically dependent on nicotine?

Not all smokers are physically dependent. Whether or not you are depends on the amount you smoke and your susceptibility to the chemical. To help you decide which quitting strategy is best for you, you must determine whether or not you are physically dependent on nicotine.

How dependent on nicotine are you?

The most common way to determine your level of dependence on nicotine is to complete the Fagenström questionnaire, which follows. This questionnaire was developed by the Swedish researcher K. O. Fagenström.

Circle the letter next to the most appropriate answer for each question.

1. How soon after you wake up do you smoke your first cigarette?
   a. after thirty minutes
   b. within thirty minutes

2. Do you find it difficult to refrain from smoking in places where it is forbidden, such as the library, theater, or doctor's office?
   a. yes
   b. no

3. Which of all the cigarettes you smoke in a day is the most satisfying?
   a. any other than the first one in the morning
   b. the first one in the morning

4. How many cigarettes do you smoke per day?
   a. 1 to 15
   b. 16 to 25
   c. 26 or more

5. Do you smoke more during the morning than during the rest of the day?
   a. yes
   b. no

6. Do you smoke when you are so ill that you are in bed most of the day?
   a. yes
   b. no

7. Does the brand you smoke have a low, medium, or high nicotine content? (Refer to your cigarette pack.)
   a. low (0.9 milligrams or less)
   b. medium (1.0 milligrams to 1.2 milligrams)
   c. high (1.3 milligrams or more)

8. How often do you inhale the smoke from your cigarette?
   a. never
   b. sometimes
   c. always

Score your answers as follows:

Question 1	0 points for a 1 point for b
Question 2	1 point for a 0 points for b
Question 3	0 points for a 1 point for b
Question 4	0 points for a 1 point for b 2 points for c
Question 5	1 point for a 0 points for b
Question 6	1 point for a 0 points for b
Question 7	0 points for a 1 point for b 2 points for c
Question 8	0 points for a 1 point for b 2 points for c

Add your total number of points. There is no passing or failing grade for this questionnaire, but higher scores indicate a higher degree of nicotine addiction. A high score (for instance, greater than 6 points) suggests that you have a very high dependence on cigarettes. For you, success in quitting will require extra effort and planning.

If you have a low score, you're in a better position to succeed. But that doesn't mean quitting will be easy. It never is. You are fortunate, however, not to be as dependent on nicotine as others. Take advantage of the opportunity to quit now, before your dependence grows.

What about the psychological dependence?

Physical dependence is only a small part of the story. It is psychological dependence on cigarettes that is to blame for the majority of failures to quit smoking. Many smokers can get past the physical discomfort of nicotine withdrawal. The hard part is to defeat the long-term craving for cigarettes.

In the past, some experts thought that physical dependence on nicotine was the primary reason that smokers had trouble quitting. Now, behavioral scientists recognize what most smokers knew all along—smoking behavior is complex and cannot be explained merely as the physical addiction to nicotine.

Your emotional dependence on cigarettes is also a very important obstacle to quitting. Physical withdrawal is unpleasant, but it passes within weeks. However, the intense craving for cigarettes, an indication of your emotional dependence, can last for years. You must learn to defeat those haunting voices in the back of your head that will plead for just one more cigarette!

You may have heard many logical arguments as to why you should stop smoking. But until now, they haven't helped you stop. Why is this so? Because your desire to continue smoking is also emotional. It is based more on an unwillingness to break the habit than on anything else. Even knowing that smoking is dangerous to your health isn't enough. Yes, medical information may have an impact on your emotional dependence upon smoking. That makes it important. But you may still ignore this practical information because of the fear of what you'll go through if you attempt to break the habit.

There are many ways in which psychological dependence can affect you. You may experience feelings that are practically impossible to distinguish from physical withdrawal. For example, you may fear that you will never regain your ability to concentrate. You may fear that you will lose your creativity, productivity, or sensitivity. These unpleasant feelings can sabotage you. In fact, you may start questioning whether or not it is really necessary to quit! The grip of your addiction may override your desire for health and long life. You may even feel that life without cigarettes can't be any fun!

How does this emotional dependence begin?

Emotional and physical dependence are closely related. The reactions a smoker has are "Pavlovian." What does this mean? Remember the psychological experiments in which Ivan Pavlov rang a bell and then fed his dogs? Soon, merely hearing a bell would make the dogs salivate. The bell had become an environmental signal associated with food. Its sound made the dogs hungry because they anticipated food.

Similarly, cigarettes can become an important part of your routine. For example, do you smoke with or after breakfast? For you, a cigarette with breakfast may have become like bacon with eggs, or milk with cereal. It may have become part of the taste, smell, and feel of the morning. This could have occurred gradually enough that you barely noticed—except that every morning, without exception, you smoke. Morning would not feel right without a cigarette.

Next, the effects of nicotine may have become not only associated with the morning but strongly tied to its smells. Your morning cup of coffee may have become linked with cigarettes. The smell of coffee triggers a strong urge for a cigarette (nicotine). Perhaps coffee at any time of day creates an urge for cigarettes.

The sights, sounds, and smells that entice you to smoke are called cues. Certain environmental cues may make it hard for you to abstain from cigarettes. The cues are your danger points. In order to succeed, you'll need to identify and overcome them.

What are common smoking cues?

Places, activities, smells, sounds, and tastes may become highly associated with cigarettes. For example, a teacher (and former smoker) recalls that the hardest part about quitting was giving up her cigarettes while she graded papers. Now, even after years of abstinence, she finds that grading papers still triggers a craving for cigarettes.

Emotions are another common category of cues. Do you smoke when you feel stressed, tired, angry, depressed, or any other such feeling? Any of these may cause a craving for cigarettes that is hard to resist.

Think about your use of tobacco. When do you use it? What is it that makes you crave it? You can probably identify some cues that push you to smoke.

How do these cues become so closely associated with smoking?

Every time you smoke, you reward yourself with a dose of nicotine. A pack-a-day smoker may take over 70,000 puffs a year. That is 70,000 annual reinforcements for the activity of smoking! No wonder it is so hard to quit. For what other activity do you reward yourself 70,000 times a year? If you've smoked for over twenty years, you will have puffed a cigarette over a 1,000,000 times! Aside from breathing, blinking, and swallowing, there are few human activities that approach this frequency. Just one cigarette in the morning at breakfast adds up to 3,650 puffs (or doses of nicotine) a year.

The cigarette also becomes associated with your self-image. This frequent activity soon becomes part of your mannerisms and appearance. You may wonder how you can be the same person without smoking. It has become more than an activity—it has become part of you.

Are there other ways in which cigarettes can produce emotional dependence?

Cigarette smoking may have strong emotional appeal to some smokers for other reasons. For many, smoking represents defiance or rebellion. It may have been an early act of independence for an adolescent. A high school student who sneaks puffs in the bathroom may view smoking as a forbidden pleasure. Smoking may continue to be an act of individuality, especially in a society that is becoming increasingly negative toward smokers.

Smoking also represents an available and easy way for some smokers to experience pleasure. This may be particularly enticing to those who feel they have little control over other aspects of their lives. Many of these smokers have difficulty even thinking about eliminating one of their few sources of enjoyment.

Advertising: External Influences

The way you feel inside is not the only factor that makes it hard to quit. You're under a lot of pressure from your environment as well. One of the major sources is the tobacco industry.

How do the tobacco companies encourage smoking habits?

Tobacco companies employ large advertising firms to shape your desire to smoke. Enormous profits are at stake. Do you consider yourself immune to the barrage of tobacco advertising that you see and hear daily? Don't underestimate the influence of Madison Avenue. Tremendous advertising resources are directed at you. In many cases, they work. You are the target of ads that portray smoking as part of the "good life." These ads associate cigarettes with youth, beauty, healthy activities, and professional success. You see these ads everywhere. They suggest that smoking is wonderful.

There are multibillion-dollar conglomerates that control most of the cigarette sales in this country. They use money, power, and sophisticated marketing techniques to keep you a smoker. Their livelihood depends on your continuing to be an addict. They want you to be unwilling, as well as unable, to stop. They put a lot of pressure on the public because, with so many smokers quitting (or dying!), they need to keep as many as possible smoking!

How much money do the tobacco companies devote to advertising each year?

The tobacco industry spends over $2 billion annually on advertising and promotions. In 1988 alone, American cigarette manufacturers spent $3.27 billion. This is the equivalent of about $100 per second! Over 20 percent of the money spent on outdoor advertising (such as billboards) is spent by tobacco companies.

The cigarette industry is closely tied to the media. It is the second leading advertiser in magazines. For example, in 1981, *Time* received over $40 million in cigarette ad revenues. In the same year, *Newsweek* received $30 million. In addition, tobacco companies are the third leading source of advertising in newspapers. In 1984, *The Washington Post* received over $2 million in cigarette ad revenues.

What are the effects of this advertising?

The major cigarette companies claim that their advertising is only meant to encourage smokers to use a particular brand. They deny that they're trying to entice people to become smokers or to discourage current smokers from quitting. They try to portray smoking as an act of freedom and associate it with democracy and free enterprise as if they are furthering the ideals of our founding fathers!

Do you see what they're really doing? These advertisers are trying to transform a dangerous, expensive, and addictive habit into a socially acceptable and politically correct way to have fun.

The ads also have an indirect effect. As newspapers and magazines depend more heavily on cigarette accounts, they may shy away from stories that place cigarettes in an unfavorable light. Furthermore, remember that all of the tobacco companies are large conglomerates that sell many products and purchase millions of dollars more in advertising. As a result, their clout is even stronger than suggested by cigarette advertising revenue alone.

Do you doubt that cigarette companies use economic force to defend their product from attack? Health-policy expert Ken Warner and his colleagues at the University of Michigan School of Public Health published an article in the *New England Journal of Medicine* in 1992 that discussed cigarette advertising and magazine coverage of the hazards of smoking. They observed that in 1988, cigarette manufacturers in the United States spent $355 million on cigarette advertising in magazines and that cigarettes were the second most heavily advertised product in magazines. In a sophisticated analysis of ninety-nine periodicals, they found that the more cigarette advertising magazines have, the less likely they are to have articles covering the hazards of smoking. This relationship was most evident in women's magazines. Warner reported that women's magazines that did not carry cigarette advertisements were more than twice as likely to have articles on the risks of smoking than were women's magazines that *did* accept cigarette advertising. Although this study did not provide proof that the dependence of these magazines on revenues from cigarette advertising has caused them to restrict their coverage of smoking and health, there are few other plausible explanations.

The clout of the tobacco companies is not limited to magazines. The cigarette manufacturers are huge conglomerates, and economic reprisals for antismoking activities can be made in many ways. For instance, in 1988, R.J. Reynolds–Nabisco cancelled an $80 million account for advertising food products with Saatchi and Saatchi, the company that prepared advertisements for the Northwest Airlines program to ban smoking on all domestic flights. On April 17, 1988, in an article titled "Tobacco Companies Turn Up the Heat on Firms Pushing Smoking Bans," *The Washington Post* reported that Walter Merryman, vice president of the Tobacco Institute (a group that represents the interests of the tobacco companies), tried to explain this action by saying, "If we are attacked, we are not going to roll over and play dead. The sooner our adversaries, friendly or otherwise, learn that, the less difficulty they are going to find themselves in."

What are the other marketing tools of these companies?

Tobacco companies are also involved in more subtle forms of promoting smoking. Promotional events are their new, powerful marketing tool. Cigarette conglomerates, by associating with high-quality events, portray themselves as a more acceptable part of society. For example, they support tennis tournaments, concerts, artistic endeavors, and professional events. They place their logos beside scoreboards, on stages, in programs, and even on athletes! Unbelievable, right? For example, when they are targeting African Americans, they sponsor events for the United Negro College Fund. To target Hispanics, they published a directory of national Hispanic organizations. When they target women, they fund women's tennis tournaments. To target youth, they support the publication of a brochure called *Helping Youth Decide* for the National Association of State Boards of Education.

Why do reputable and respected organizations associate their projects with the tobacco industry? It's simple. They need the money. The economic power of the cigarette companies is used to try to buy respectability. The companies attempt to portray themselves as benefactors. For them, this is certainly more advantageous than being seen as promoting a deadly activity that leads to almost 400,000 deaths a year! Consider the irony of these tobacco company-sponsored events. For instance, a tobacco company sponsors the Kool Jazz Festival even though smoking has been responsible for the deaths of many chain-smoking jazz greats, including Duke Ellington, who died of lung cancer.

PSYCHOLOGICAL OBSTACLES TO QUITTING

In addition to the internal and external influences that make it hard to quit, there are a number of obstacles that can make quitting even more difficult. How many of these concern you?

Obstacle 1: Fear of Failure

Have you thought about quitting but haven't done anything about it because you were afraid of failure? If so, you're not alone. This is a very common obstacle. Everyone knows that it's hard to quit, and no one wants to fail.

Not only may you be concerned about your failure, but you might also worry about what others will think of you if you do fail! This may be an especially important concern if you have attempted to quit many times before. Quitting can be a very public event, as many people become aware that you are making the attempt. As a result, the prospect of failure becomes even more scary.

What should you do? Restructure your thinking to take on a more positive, constructive attitude. You deserve credit for moving from "not thinking about quitting" to "thinking about quitting" to "doing something about it." This is a step in the right direction. But what happens if you do get stalled at that point?

Don't look at it as if you have failed. Rather, remember that quitting is a process of change. It takes some smokers longer than others to complete the process. The goal of this book is to help you accelerate your progress to achieve success. In order to continue along that path, you should focus on the partial success you achieve in every effort you make.

Are you discouraged by prior failures? Many smokers are and find this to be another major obstacle. But previous failure does *not* have to be an indicator of how you will do this time. (And you've never had this book before, have you?)

A smoker's failure to stop has been studied extensively. Research has shown that with each attempt to quit, you're actually starting with a clean slate. What you really want to do, as long as you're starting over, is to undertake strategies that will increase your chances of success. If you do this, it is inevitable that you will eventually succeed. There is *no one* who cannot ultimately succeed in quitting cigarettes—as long as he or she really wants to.

Let's conclude our discussion of this obstacle with a little pep talk. You're reading this book because you want to succeed at quitting, right? Don't let yourself be stymied by concerns about failure. You are not helpless. You have the power to take control back from nicotine. You can succeed. Your path to victory may have some ups and downs, but eventually you will free yourself from cigarettes. There is only one way to guarantee you'll remain a smoker for your entire life and that is to refuse to do anything to stop!

Obstacle 2: Concerns About Weight Gain

Are you afraid to stop smoking because you don't want to gain weight? The potential for weight gain presents an important obstacle to many smokers. This may be a significant problem for you. It can certainly test your determination to quit. Do you fit into this category? If so, the best way to confront these concerns is to know the facts.

Will you gain weight after you quit smoking?

Many people gain a little weight each year as a matter of course. If you quit smoking, you may gain more than you would have if you had continued to smoke. Studies of weight changes in smokers who quit show that almost eight in ten will gain weight over a two-year period. This statistic sounds alarmingly high. But guess what? More than five in ten of the people who *continue* to smoke gain weight anyway. Therefore, although giving up cigarettes does increase the risk of weight gain, it doesn't guarantee it.

Whether or not you will gain weight is really hard to predict. There is very little known about which smokers have the greatest risk of adding pounds after quitting. Some people, however, do have a propensity to gain. If you have quit before, then you probably have a better idea of whether or not this affects you.

How much weight will you gain?

The real problem with gaining weight is not whether you'll gain but how much! Relax. Here are the facts. Smokers who quit do gain a little more weight than smokers who continue. Research has shown that over a two-year period after quitting, successful quitters gain an average of five pounds. But the people who keep smoking gain about one pound in the same time period. Therefore, despite all the concerns you probably have about this, the average weight gain as a result of quitting is only four pounds more than would be expected if you continued smoking. (Of course, you will have something to do with that!)

Your greatest concern is probably that you would gain significantly. Most people are not disturbed by the thought of gaining five pounds but become distraught at the thought of gaining ten to twenty! In a two-year study of almost 10,000 quitters and smokers, however, only a very small percentage gained twenty pounds during this period. About 4 in 100 of the people who quit gained twenty pounds, as compared to 1 in 100 who continued to smoke. So, yes, there were more quitters who gained a significant amount of weight, but it was a very small percentage.

What causes weight gain after quitting?

Scientists do not understand precisely why smokers have a tendency to weigh less than people who do not smoke. One thought is that they often smoke instead of eating, thereby consuming less food. Many studies support this idea. For instance, one study found that smokers who quit increased their daily food consumption by about 200 calories (equal to approximately one candy bar). This may not sound like a large amount, but it could account for much of the reported weight increase.

Another important cause of weight gain is the effect of cigarettes on your metabolism. Metabolism refers to your overall use of energy. Food provides energy to your body. If your body is very efficient (uses energy conservatively) and requires a small amount of fuel (sounds like a car, doesn't it?), then extra energy will turn into fat and be stored as such. Smoking may make your body less efficient and increase your metabolic rate. The decrease in your metabolic rate after quitting may be the most important contributor to the accompanying weight gain.

What can you do to prevent weight gain?

Increased weight is *not* an inevitable consequence of smoking cessation. Many people do not even gain one pound after quitting. Paying attention to your diet and exercising can counteract any tendency you might have to gain. (We'll discuss this more in a later section.) Learning to focus on a healthier lifestyle may complement your attempt to quit smoking.

There are currently no good medical approaches to the problem of mild weight gain after smoking cessation. Nevertheless, there is some evidence that nicotine is the agent in cigarette smoke that contributes to lower body weight. Therefore, replacement of nicotine would seem to be a natural treatment of both smoke cessation and weight gain. Small-scale studies have suggested that nicotine gum can decrease or eliminate the problem. The use of other medications should be avoided. No current medication has shown promise as an aid to controlling weight without causing significant side effects. If there were such a medication, you would have heard about it.

What should you do about weight-gain concerns?

The first thing to do when concerns about weight gain throw an obstacle in your path is to accept the fact that some weight gain is possible but to remember that it usually involves only a few pounds. In addition, you can plan to lose any extra weight after you have quit. Right now, giving up smoking is more beneficial to you than avoiding the possibility of gaining a few pounds. That's our recommendation.

Once you make the decision that you want to quit smoking, the best strategy is to focus all of your attention on achieving your goal. You can try to minimize any weight gain by paying attention to your food intake and level of exercise. Reassure yourself that any problems with weight gain that you do experience will be dealt with later. Concede that you may add some pounds, but remind yourself that it is more important that you quit smoking. Most importantly, don't allow any concerns about weight gain to lead to a rationalization that you shouldn't quit.

Obstacle 3: Concerns About Loss of Productivity

Do you believe that smoking helps you think and concentrate? If so, you're probably concerned that your mental performance will suffer if you stop. You might even consider cigarette smoking to be vital to your work and worry that your productivity will decrease if you quit. This concern is sufficient to keep some smokers from making the attempt.

What is the connection between smoking and mental performance?

Some smokers think that smoking enhances their ability to concentrate, improves their memory, and augments their problem-solving abilities. Whether or not cigarettes really have this power is far from clear. This question has been the subject of many studies. No doubt you have your own beliefs about the role of cigarettes in your mental performance. If you are a moderate to heavy smoker, you probably feel that they do make some contribution.

Is there evidence that smoking increases your ability to concentrate?

Researchers have examined this question by having smokers

(while smoking and not smoking) and nonsmokers perform repetitive tasks that require concentration. In these studies, the
nonsmokers tended to do better than the smokers, both with and
without cigarettes. But several studies showed that some smokers
actually did a little better on these tests while smoking. Why?
Smokers who were not allowed to smoke may have been thinking
about cigarettes, which may have distracted them from the task.
So maybe it's not that cigarettes increase concentration but that
taking them away actually decreases it. In sum, although certain
studies suggest a connection between smoking and attention,
performance, and concentration, no definitive conclusions can be
drawn.

Does smoking improve your learning ability?

Some studies suggest that learning is enhanced by smoking. Other
studies strongly disagree with this notion. So you'll get no definitive answer on this one either. However, anticipate that your
ability to concentrate may be impaired as you withdraw from
cigarettes. Why? You may be easily distracted and might even feel
slightly disoriented. But as you get through the first week or so,
this should pass. After a short period of time, you should notice
that there is no perceptible difference in your mental performance.

Obstacle 4: Concerns About Stress

Do you use cigarettes to deal with stressful situations? Many
smokers report that they do. Some studies suggest that nicotine is
helpful in improving moods and decreasing negative feelings
during stressful times. Why this occurs is not well understood, but
it may explain why you like to smoke at these times.

   If you use smoking to cope with stressful situations, then the
idea of quitting may be frightening and may even be sufficient to
prevent you from quitting. Of course, smoking to relieve stress is
not the answer. Sure, smoking may be helpful to you in this way,
but at what cost? Wouldn't it be better to find ways that do not
harm you?

   So, again, you are confronted with a personal decision. If you
use smoking for stress reduction, you must make the decision that

you will find other ways to cope. Once you decide that this is important to you, then you can do it.

As long as we're talking about stress, what about the stress of quitting, which for some people can be very stressful? Not everyone experiences this. There is a widespread belief that giving up cigarettes is always an emotionally trying experience. Some people do describe the first weeks as torture. Sure, quitting may be difficult. But please don't anticipate that giving up smoking is going to be a psychologically damaging experience. Studies show that quitting cigarettes does not drive people to alcohol or mental breakdowns. Yes, quitting is challenging, but it won't be damaging to your mental stability. You are not sacrificing your mental fitness to improve your physical well-being. What you want is to reduce stress more appropriately and develop more positive ways to cope. We'll discuss how to do this later.

Obstacle 5: Concerns About Nicotine Withdrawal

The more you expose your body to nicotine, the more your body needs it and the less it responds to it. This phenomenon occurs with many addictive substances. It's part of the addictive triad we mentioned earlier. How do you know you're physically dependent? You can judge by the reaction of your body when it is deprived of nicotine, even for a brief period. At that time, lack of nicotine sets off a withdrawal syndrome.

Some smokers are reluctant to act on their desire to quit because of concerns about nicotine withdrawal. You might be concerned that quitting will cause you a lot of unpleasantness. This fear should not deter you from action for a few reasons. Withdrawal is not as bad as it is often portrayed. Some people don't have any physical withdrawal symptoms. And even if you do experience some, they usually last only for a week or so. Finally, there are ways to effectively deal with nicotine withdrawal if you are one of the people for whom it is troublesome.

What is the best way to cope with withdrawal? Learn what to expect. It always helps to understand what is happening to your body. Of course, if you have tried to quit before, then you're probably an expert on how your body reacts to nicotine withdrawal.

What exactly happens during nicotine withdrawal?

Nicotine withdrawal is described in medical books as a syndrome resulting from the abrupt cessation or reduction of the use of nicotine-containing substances that have been employed for at least a moderate duration and in moderate amounts. As we discussed, when you withdraw from nicotine by giving up cigarettes, your heart rate may slow, your blood pressure may rise, and you may experience other physiological and psychological reactions. In order for you to be medically diagnosed with nicotine withdrawal, now called tobacco withdrawal syndrome, you must meet the following criteria:

• Daily use of nicotine for at least several weeks

• Abrupt cessation or reduction of nicotine followed within twenty-four hours by at least four of the following symptoms:
   —craving for nicotine
   —irritability, frustration, or anger
   —anxiety
   —difficulty concentrating
   —restlessness
   —decreased heart rate
   —increased appetite or weight gain

Have you met these criteria? If so, you've suffered from nicotine withdrawal. Some people have reported depression, disrupted sleep, impatience, impaired work performance, and increased enjoyment of sweets as well. Cigarette craving is the most commonly experienced symptom. Psychological withdrawal symptoms are unpleasant, it's true. But, remember, they don't last!

When does withdrawal begin and how long does it persist?

If you're going to experience withdrawal symptoms, they usually peak in intensity during the first twenty-four to forty-eight hours after you stop using nicotine. Fortunately for most smokers, the physical symptoms do not last long and diminish within two weeks. For some, the symptoms disappear within two weeks; others, however, complain about irritability or difficulty concentrating for a lot longer. Psychological cravings, usually the cause of these difficulties, can last much longer.

Can you have withdrawal symptoms while you sleep?

As was previously mentioned, when you smoke, nicotine rapidly enters your bloodstream and stays in your body for many hours. If you smoke frequently during the day, enough nicotine can accumulate in your body to last through the night. This is why many smokers who are physically dependent on nicotine light up soon after waking in the morning. They start the day with a low level of nicotine in their blood, and need even more to awaken fully and to avoid those unpleasant withdrawal symptoms.

Does every smoker suffer a withdrawal syndrome when they quit?

Not everyone experiences withdrawal symptoms. You may be lucky and, despite years of smoking, not have any. Statistically, about one in four heavy smokers and most light smokers experience no symptoms. Whether or not you will can't be accurately predicted simply from the number of cigarettes you smoke. Nor can you predict how severe the symptoms will be. Why? One reason may be that people who smoke the same number of cigarettes may consume very different amounts of nicotine because of the way they smoke. Your daily nicotine intake depends on the following: the number of cigarettes you smoke; the type of cigarettes; how deeply you inhale; how many puffs of each cigarette you take; how much of each cigarette you smoke; and even how you hold the cigarette!

How do we know that nicotine accounts for withdrawal symptoms?

The exact same symptoms are seen in all heavy users of nicotine when they go for a while without the substance. It does not matter if you get your nicotine from cigarettes, chewing tobacco, or snuff. Nicotine is a drug, and you'll feel the same unpleasant symptoms no matter which form you consumed it in. Similarly, these symptoms can promptly be relieved by taking nicotine in any form. (That's why so many smokers return to their habits.)

What can you do about withdrawal?

Since nicotine is the cause of withdrawal symptoms, it can also be used to treat them. This is where nicotine replacements, in the form of gum, patches, or spray, have been used. (This subject is discussed in detail in Chapter 5.) Why is this important? It's good for you to know that there are products available that can effectively blunt or reduce the symptoms of nicotine withdrawal. This can be the difference between success and failure in quitting. So you should not allow concerns about withdrawal to prevent you from giving up cigarettes.

Obstacle 6: Concerns About Your Age

Many older smokers feel discouraged about quitting because they believe they are too old to change their ways and too old to benefit. In a recent survey of people over sixty-five who were thinking about quitting, two-thirds were not confident that they could succeed. Almost half of the smokers over sixty-five reported that they did not believe quitting would provide them with health benefits, and an almost equal number did not believe that continuing to smoke would harm them. If you're in this age group and if that is what you believe, then it's easy to understand the difficulty you might have in being motivated to quit.

The facts combat this obstacle well. Many older Americans have successfully quit smoking. You do not stop being able to make constructive changes in your life when you grow older. Even if you have been physically unaffected by smoking until now, you're still at high risk for the unhealthy consequences if you continue. Among older smokers, the benefits of smoking cessation, such as reducing the chances of heart disease and stroke, occur almost immediately.

SUMMARY

Unfortunately, you can always find reasons not to quit. There are certainly plenty of obstacles to your success. However, if you can identify these obstacles, then you can triumph over them. At this point, the most important thing to do is to convince yourself that, despite the challenges, quitting is worth the effort! Take a deep breath and move from contemplation to action. The next chapter begins the action stage. Are you ready to actively prepare for success? Good. Let's move on.

CHAPTER 3

Building a Foundation for Success

To increase your chances of quitting, you need to build a strong foundation for success. What can you do to create this foundation? There are a few important preparation strategies that should be part of every smoker's plan for quitting. Let's discuss them in detail.

LEARN ABOUT SMOKING

You are an expert about smoking. You know how it makes you feel. You know how much pleasure you get from it, which brands you like, and that smoking is not good for your health. At first, the idea of learning about smoking may seem like an unnecessary part of preparing to quit. Wrong! It is not only necessary, it is also crucial.

Why is it so important to learn about smoking? Because understanding smoking as an addiction is critical to investigating and implementing ways to free yourself from cigarettes. Knowledge about smoking demystifies cigarettes. Seeing them as merely a way to deliver doses of nicotine to your brain makes them less attractive. Reading about the motives of multibillion dollar advertising campaigns by the tobacco companies provides insight into the ways the public can be manipulated for private gain.

Research has suggested that more people give up smoking because of what they expect the benefits to be when they stop than because they simply are afraid of continuing. Therefore, you want to emphasize the benefits you will derive when you become an ex-smoker. This strategy increases your likelihood of ongoing success.

What are the two main benefits that most people see as reasons for quitting? They are improvements in health and increased confidence in handling stressful situations without cigarettes.

Where does all the information about smoking come from? It has been obtained as a result of decades of research by dedicated scientists who spend your tax dollars. So as long as you have paid for it, why not put this wealth of information to work for you!

BELIEVE IN YOURSELF—YOU CAN QUIT SMOKING

> "I think I can, I think I can, I think I can. . . ."
> —from *The Little Engine That Could*

Believing in yourself is not only important, it is also essential for success. Most smokers who successfully quit have the belief and expectation that they can make this change.

You *can* quit smoking. Quitting may be difficult, but it is not an impossible task. Much research has demonstrated that the power of cigarettes can be overcome. Almost 50 percent of the people who report ever having smoked have quit. About fifty years ago, nearly half the population of the United States smoked. It was almost an expected ritual of adulthood. In contrast, today only about 25 percent of the population smokes.

As we mentioned in Chapter 1, many people try to quit several times before they are ultimately successful. Many people who succeed do so because they try a number of techniques in combination. In other words, if you use a number of different quit-smoking strategies together, you may increase the likelihood that you will triumph.

But remember, regardless of what techniques you use, you must be committed to stopping. You must believe that you can stop.

There are a number of factors that can increase the likelihood of your success, but you must first be motivated to quit. Once you have this motivation, you'll then want to turn it into a fruitful action plan.

In order to minimize the fear or anticipation of failure, recognize that even though you may have tried before, and you may be discouraged, there are many others like you who have been successful.

INVESTIGATE WHY YOU SMOKE

Smokers usually have many different reasons for smoking. These range from pure pleasure to relaxation to control or reduction of stress to simply fulfilling a habit. The same smoker may sometimes smoke for different reasons.

There are a number of reasons why people start and continue smoking even though they know it is not in their best interest to do so.

Smoking as a Self-Indulgence

People tend to smoke because they feel they are doing something that they want to do. This may be in contrast to the pressures of life, which often make people feel that they are not able to do any of the things they enjoy. Because of this, they are often reluctant to give up one of the few things that is readily available to them. Whether or not you have difficulties socially, vocationally, personally, or physically, smoking can be a constant source of self-indulgent "pleasure." This may be stronger than any practical reasons for stopping.

Smoking as a Stress Reducer

Many people care less about the taste of smoking than they do about the feeling of relaxation that they get from it. We know, physiologically, that smoking is not a relaxant. However, the psychological relaxation benefits are significant and well-documented.

The pressures of everyday life can be exorbitant. People tend to grasp at anything that can reliably and consistently help them reduce pressure and stress. By smoking, you can engage in a behavior that, even for a brief period of time, gives you an excuse to take a break. You don't have to be concerned about a boss or someone looking at you and wondering why you're sitting and doing nothing. Your justification is that you're in the process of lighting up. Therefore, anything that may be asked of you is put on hold for that short period of time. Further, if you're talking to people and you don't know what to say, taking a drag of a cigarette can be a momentary respite.

You can also relax by smoking simply because of the deep breathing that is required. Deep breathing, which by its very nature is calming, is more a part of the smoking process than is normal breathing. Research indicates that smokers take more deep breaths than nonsmokers.

Smoking can also be relaxing because it's nice to anticipate. Isn't it comforting to look forward to something that will provide a few moments of pleasure? Stress and the world around you are briefly put aside. You can focus exclusively on something you enjoy.

Smoking as a Way of Avoiding Withdrawal

As we discussed in Chapter 2, some people continue smoking simply because they're afraid of withdrawal symptoms. Depending on who you ask, you'll find out that withdrawal is anything ranging from "no big deal" to "the worst experience of my (and my family's) life!" So it's easy to understand how fear of withdrawal may "motivate" someone to keep smoking.

Smoking as a Social Booster

Many people find it difficult to interact comfortably with others. Smoking may help smooth over awkward moments. For example, what if you're not sure how to communicate or what to do with your hands or body while you're talking? Smoking can give you an excuse; it can distract, or otherwise occupy, you. Cigarettes can be a prop or tool to help you feel more comfortable.

In a social situation, smoking may make you feel more confident. You may feel more mature, sophisticated, or worldly because you are engaged in an "adult" behavior. Of course, it seems ironic to consider something that is damaging to your health as being mature!

Smoking as a Weight Controller

As we explained in the previous chapter, many people smoke because they feel it keeps their weight down. They may have tried to quit smoking previously and found that their weight increased. Or maybe they read that people gain weight by quitting and they're reluctant to have this happen. In addition, they may believe that if they use cigarettes instead of eating when they are hungry, they will eat less. That can keep their weight under control. Physiologically, cigarettes do suppress appetite to a small degree, leading some people to maintain smoking as a weight-controlling behavior. Further, smoking can alter your ability to taste foods. This may also contribute to keeping your weight down, since if you're less able to taste foods, you may have less of a desire to eat.

Smoking as a Pleasant Physical Activity

Many people like the way handling a cigarette feels. It gives them something to do with their hands (and their mouths). By having something physical to do, they may momentarily be distracted from something that is stressful or consuming.

REVIEWING THE REASONS
FOR CONTINUING TO SMOKE

All of the reasons just mentioned have one common theme. They are all perceived as being positive reasons to continue smoking. This makes the act of stopping that much more difficult. If the only results of smoking were negative, it would be a lot easier to stop. For example, if you put your hand over an open flame, it hurts, you get burned, and you get scared. There are no positive reasons to continue, so you don't. With smoking, however, people feel there *are* positive reasons to continue.

What should be your main goal right now? Recognize that any and all of the positive values you get from smoking can be achieved through nonsmoking behaviors. We'll talk later about learning to do just that.

KNOW THYSELF

People smoke for many different reasons. It's important for you to understand exactly why you smoke. This will help you in your efforts to stop. Sure, you say, but I have lived with myself, so I already know what my smoking habits are. But study the things that you do and your reasons for smoking. By doing so, not only will you learn additional information that may be helpful in your stop-smoking campaign, but you will also commit yourself to the process of stopping.

Ask yourself questions about your smoking. Make sure you write down the answers. These questions should be helpful in determining why and how you smoke. Such questions should include how long you have smoked, how many cigarettes per day you smoke, and at what times during the day you smoke.

Have you ever stopped smoking? If so, using what programs? How well did the programs work? Why didn't they succeed? Who are the significant people around you who also smoke? What types of cigarettes do you like? Where do you keep them? What are the triggers for your smoking behavior? What are the consequences, both positive and negative, of your smoking?

There are two key strategies you can use to learn about your smoking behavior: complete the following questionnaire, and monitor your smoking behavior carefully.

The National Cancer Institute Questionnaire

An understanding of what motivates you to smoke can help you select an appropriate strategy to quit. By learning why you smoke, you can attack the underlying causes. This is an opportunity to take better control of smoking—and your life!

Why Do You Smoke?

Directions: Here are some statements made by people to describe what they get out of smoking cigarettes. How often do you feel this way when smoking? Circle one number for each statement. Important: answer every question.

	always	frequently	sometimes	seldom	never
A. I smoke cigarettes in order to keep myself from slowing down.	5	4	3	2	1
B. Handling a cigarette is part of the enjoyment of smoking it.	5	4	3	2	1
C. Smoking cigarettes is pleasant and relaxing.	5	4	3	2	1
D. I light up a cigarette when I feel angry about something.	5	4	3	2	1
E. When I have run out of cigarettes, I find it almost unbearable until I can get them.	5	4	3	2	1
F. I smoke cigarettes automatically without even being aware of it.	5	4	3	2	1
G. I smoke cigarettes to stimulate me, to perk myself up.	5	4	3	2	1
H. Part of the enjoyment of smoking a cigarette comes from the steps I take to light up.	5	4	3	2	1
I. I find cigarettes pleasurable.	5	4	3	2	1
J. When I feel uncomfortable or upset about something, I light up a cigarette.	5	4	3	2	1
K. I am very much aware of the fact when I am notsmoking a cigarette.	5	4	3	2	1
L. I light up a cigarette without realizing I still have one burning in the ashtray.	5	4	3	2	1
M. I smoke cigarettes to give me a "lift."	5	4	3	2	1
N. When I smoke a cigarette, part of the enjoyment is watching the smoke as I exhale it.	5	4	3	2	1
O. I want a cigarette most when I am comfortable and relaxed.	5	4	3	2	1
P. When I feel blue or want to take my mind off cares and worries, I smoke cigarettes.	5	4	3	2	1
Q. I get a real gnawing hunger for a cigarette when I haven't smoked for a while.	5	4	3	2	1
R. I've found a cigarette in my mouth and didn't remember putting it there.	5	4	3	2	1

How to Score

1. Enter the number you have circled for each question in the spaces below, putting the number you have circled to question A over line A, to question B over line B, etc.

2. Add the three scores on each line to get your totals. For example, the sum of your scores over lines A, G, and M gives you your score on Stimulation—lines B, H, and N give the score on Handling, etc.

Totals

___		___		___	
A	+	G	+	M	=

___ Stimulation

___		___		___	
B	+	H	+	N	=

___ Handling

___		___		___	
C	+	I	+	O	=

___ Pleasurable Relaxation

___		___		___	
D	+	J	+	P	=

___ Crutch: Tension Reduction

___		___		___	
E	+	K	+	Q	=

___ Craving: Psychological Addiction

___		___		___	
F	+	L	+	R	=

___ Habit

Scores can vary from 3 to 15. Any score 11 and above is high; any score 7 and below is low.

These questions are designed to help you clarify why you smoke. They describe six different reasons. The first three focus on the positive feelings that people derive from cigarettes. Reason number one is the stimulation that a cigarette provides. A high score on this category suggests that you like feeling stimulated by cigarettes. You enjoy it and feel it boosts your energy.

Handling a cigarette is the second reason that some people smoke. You might get a positive feeling from holding a cigarette. You like the rituals involved in smoking—tamping, lighting, dragging, and so on. You enjoy watching the smoke come out of your nose, or blowing smoke rings.

You may like the feeling of relaxation provided by smoking. This is the third reason. It may have become an important crutch— one you use in a variety of situations.

Strategies to help you if any of these reasons apply include: exercising, stretching, deep breathing, doodling, taking a walk, working on a hobby, knitting, taking a shower, or doing a crossword puzzle. All of these strategies try to substitute a positive behavior for smoking so you can replace the pleasures you derive from cigarettes. It may also be helpful to counteract the pleasurable feelings of smoking by focusing on the high physical cost to your body.

The other three are the negative reasons that people smoke. Reason number four is to decrease bad feelings like tension, stress, anxiety, or other discomforts. If you do this, you're actually using cigarettes as a psychological tranquilizer. However, as you probably already know, tranquilizers are not really the answer and can be fairly ineffective with long-term use. If this is why you smoke, now is the time to learn how to decrease the stress in your life as well as to find better methods of coping with tense circumstances.

Craving is another important reason that people smoke. This addictive feeling is defined as an incredibly strong desire or urge to smoke. Virtually everyone who smokes is familiar with the feeling. "I just have to have a cigarette!" they say. You may feel something is missing if you're not smoking. This craving may be a response to nicotine withdrawal, even if your body was only recently exposed to nicotine. For some reason, the nicotine level in your body may have dropped. Your body will then send you a strong message to replenish the supply.

The final reason is that some people smoke without thinking much about it. These smokers are locked into the habit. Strategies for them may be directed toward both increasing their awareness of smoking and breaking their bad habit.

Self-Monitoring

The second step for learning about your smoking behavior is to monitor it carefully. How well do you know your smoking habits? You may be unaware of the number of puffs you take, how deeply you puff, or even how many cigarettes you smoke.

It can be very helpful (and even enlightening) to keep a careful log of the cigarettes that you smoke. Take a sheet of paper that has twenty-four lines and label each line with an hour of the day. Whenever you smoke, write on the appropriate line the exact time of day, where you are, and why you smoked. Keep this log for at least a week. Then review it to see what patterns emerge.

This exercise is useful to identify your trouble spots during the day. It is also helpful in getting you to think about each cigarette. During the time that you keep the log, you will not smoke as a reflex. Why? Because with each cigarette, you'll have to think about why you are smoking.

Part II
Quit-Smoking Strategies

CHAPTER 4

Selecting Your Quit-Smoking Program

There are many different methods available today to help you stop smoking. There are literally dozens and dozens of stop-smoking programs, methods, and techniques on the market. This book would be very short if there were one smoking program that was best for every smoker. But none of them works for everyone. All of them have been successful for some individuals. One of the most important ingredients for success in virtually any program you select is that you be committed to quitting. If you're not, it doesn't matter what program you try. You will not succeed.

Since planning is the most important step to successful action, your goals must now involve comparing programs. Unfortunately, there are many methods, programs, devices, and gimmicks, and few ways to distinguish them. This makes it difficult for you to choose wisely from among the many options. But choose wisely you must, because that's what maximizes your chances for success. You'll want to learn as much as you can to make the best personal decision. What should you look for? What should you ask about? This chapter will give you some things to think about as you go through the process of determining what program is best suited to you.

COMPARING PROGRAMS

The best way to compare programs would be to find out for each one the percentage of people who successfully quit smoking out of all who attempted. That sounds easy enough. But, in practice, this is very difficult. First, many organizations and companies do not know the success rates of their programs. Others who know their rates may be reluctant to make them public. It might be felt that low success rates will discourage smokers. This can be a problem when the creators of honest programs have to compete with the claims of dishonest competitors.

Each program should be able to quote you a success rate. If one doesn't, be wary. Unless you're asking about a new program that is in the process of being evaluated, we would probably recommend that you avoid the program or technique.

COLD TURKEY VERSUS TAPERING

Research indicates there are two basic ways to stop smoking—either immediately (cold turkey) or gradually (tapering). The different programs you'll be reading about use one of these two approaches. So you'll have to decide not only what program to use but also how quickly you want to stop.

There are pros and cons to each approach. If you stop cold turkey, you're done smoking. All of your energy goes into maintenance—remaining a nonsmoker. But you may experience more symptoms of withdrawal. And cold turkey can be terrifying. To be a smoker one minute and not be allowed to have a cigarette the next can cause a panicky reaction. But many smokers (as well as many experts in the field) feel it's really the only way to succeed.

On the other hand, tapering appears to be easier. You're not stopping all at once, so withdrawal symptoms can be minimized. However, it may be harder to get rid of that last cigarette. In addition, some critics feel that tapering makes it much easier to slide back into old smoking habits.

To begin, you may want to first decide if you prefer to stop cold turkey or gradually. Then, pick a program that incorporates the chosen approach. Or you may want to select the program that most appeals to you and then follow whatever approach it uses.

ADDITIONAL FACTORS TO CONSIDER

Now let's discuss some of the additional factors that you'll want to take into account when selecting the best program for you.

When asking about success rates, you'll also want to consider issues such as timing, methods of follow-up and counting, and type of participants.

Timing

Even when program success rates are quoted, companies often neglect to tell you when these rates were determined. What is most important for you to know? The *long-term* success rate of a program. After all, what good is a program if it helps most of its participants stop smoking, but the quitters begin smoking again within three days of completion? Unfortunately, this information may not be available for many programs.

Follow-Up

You should know how success rates were determined. The rates may be inflated. Why? Often, this information is obtained by interviews, and some people may be too embarrassed to admit that they've gone back to smoking again. Also, as far as statistics are concerned, you should learn how the program dealt with participants who could not be found or who dropped out of the program. Participants who didn't return phone calls or who quit the program probably went back to smoking. Statistics that ignore these people will probably offer inflated and inaccurate success rates.

The Participants

Wouldn't you like to know something about who participated in the program? Were they heavy or light smokers? How motivated were they? Were they like you? In other words, would their results give you an idea of how successful you might be?

Success rates may give you a glimpse of a program's value, but you should also ask, "Compared to what?" In the best studies, smokers are divided randomly among two or more different programs and then followed closely to determine their success. Success rates are most useful when they can be compared between similar groups.

So where does this leave you? There is no easy answer to the question, "Is this program effective?" It is important for you to learn about the programs that interest you, find out if they make sense to you, and determine whether or not they have the endorsement of respected organizations in your community. Finally, you have to be comfortable with whatever program or technique you select. This factor, although vague, is probably the most critical one for your success.

The remaining chapters in Part II of this book will provide you with information about the methods available to help you quit smoking.

CHAPTER 5

The Nicotine-Replacement Strategy

Conquering Nicotine Dependence

We previously discussed the fact that nicotine addiction is one of the main reasons for a smoker's inability to quit. This addiction can be physiological, psychological, or both. If your nicotine addiction is physiological, the short-term replacement of nicotine in your body by a method other than smoking may be the answer.

Nicotine-replacement strategies use items other than cigarettes to replace the nicotine in your body in order to help ease your physical withdrawal from cigarettes. With this method, you'll be much more comfortable when you quit smoking.

There are four methods of nicotine replacement. The first one, smokeless tobacco, is dangerous. The second, lobeline tablets, does not work very well. Only the nicotine gum and the nicotine patch are approved by the Food and Drug Administration (FDA) as aids to smoking cessation. Let's discuss these methods, as well as some methods currently under development.

SMOKELESS TOBACCO

The oral use of smokeless tobacco, usually in the form of chewing tobacco or snuff, is the worst type of nicotine replacement that a smoker can choose. With it, you do avoid tar, carbon monoxide, and the other components of smoke, but you leave yourself open to many other risks. The *1986 Surgeon General's Report* was devoted to smokeless tobacco and concluded that it represents a significant health risk and is not a safe substitute for smoking cigarettes.

History

Chewing tobacco and snuff were popular far before cigarette smoking came into vogue. In fact, there is evidence that Native Americans chewed tobacco to alleviate hunger pangs more than 5,000 years ago! The use of snuff in the United States was documented as early as the 1600s in the Jamestown Colony. It peaked in the nineteenth century and then declined as cigarettes became popular. Nevertheless, more than 12 million Americans currently use smokeless tobacco.

Preparation

Chewing tobacco is typically held in the cheek or lower lip. Snuff is much finer in consistency than chewing tobacco. It is usually placed in the mouth but not chewed. Tobacco sniffing is rare today.

There are many different types of smokeless tobacco. These products differ in where they are grown and cultivated, in which parts of the tobacco plant are used, in the method of curing, in moisture content, and in additives. In addition, some tobaccos contain flavorings like licorice, mint, or wintergreen.

Nicotine Exposure

Even though these tobacco products are smokeless, they contain substantial quantities of nicotine. Since nicotine can be absorbed well in your mouth, the exposure to nicotine from smokeless tobacco is equivalent to that of cigarettes. Consequently, the addiction produced by this level and frequency of nicotine intake is also similar to that of cigarette smoking.

Harms

What is the major reason that smokeless tobacco is not a reasonable alternative to cigarettes? Its use greatly increases the risk of cancer. There is evidence that the risks of cancer of the mouth, nose, esophagus, voice box, and stomach are increased by using smokeless tobacco.

Effectiveness

Smokeless tobacco might seem to be a possible substitute for cigarettes, but you'll derive very little benefit from such a switch. Not only would you remain addicted to nicotine, but also your health would continue to be endangered by your use of tobacco and its carcinogenic ingredients.

Recommendation

Avoid smokeless tobacco products.

LOBELINE

Lobeline is a nicotine-like substance currently marketed as an over-the-counter smoking substitute that can be found at almost every drug store. Usually, in the aisle that contains the tobacco products, there are tablets containing lobeline sulfate that are touted as aids to smoking cessation.

History

Lobeline, discovered in 1915, is not a new product. Even before the health consequences of smoking were known for certain, there were people who wanted to quit. This substance has been used as a quitting aid since the 1930s, when lobeline capsules were first sold to decrease cigarette withdrawal symptoms. Over the years, lobeline has been taken either alone or in combination with other medicines, in the form of tablets, lozenges, or injection. (The injection, however, produces frequent gastric intestinal distress.) Lobeline is sold over-the-counter and through clinics, although by now, it has been abandoned by most legitimate clinics.

Preparation

Like nicotine, this substance is obtained from tobacco, but from a different type than that used in smoking products. Chemists describe lobeline as a less potent form of nicotine. It is marketed by many companies and under several trade names. For example, it might be found as Bantron tablets (by the JMI-Dep Corporation) or as CigArrest tablets or gum (by the Advantage Health and Fitness Corporation). The tablets usually contain 2 milligrams of lobeline and the gum contains .6 milligrams.

Effectiveness

The problem with lobeline, unlike nicotine gum (to be discussed next), is that there is no evidence that it helps anyone quit smoking. As a cigarette substitute, it does not seem to decrease cravings or increase rates of success.

The best thing that can be said about lobeline is that it does not appear to be harmful. The FDA has classified it as safe but not effective. High doses of lobeline, however, can cause abdominal pain, heartburn, nausea, and vomiting.

Recommendation

Although lobeline can be found in most drug stores as a quit-smoking aid, there is no scientific evidence to support its use. You should save your money and avoid products made with it.

NICOTINE GUM AND PATCH

In the past decade, delivery of nicotine in ways other than through tobacco has emerged as an important method to help smokers quit. Currently, nicotine polacrilex chewing gum and the nicotine skin patch are the main methods of nicotine replacement that are approved by the FDA as aids to smoking cessation.

You may have concerns about replacing one form of addiction with another. First of all, the gum and patch are designed to be used for a short time. You're not supposed to use them indefinitely. Most people can cut back on the gum or the patch gradually. A small percentage, though, will want to continue to use them. This is not recommended. But it is usually easier to help someone quit the gum or the patch than to quit smoking.

Secondly, while it is true that there is some addictive potential to nicotine gum and the patch, it is much less so than that to cigarettes. Neither the gum nor the patch creates dependence. Rather, each transfers dependence on nicotine to a different source.

You also may have concerns about exposing yourself to nicotine. Although nicotine has many effects on the body, its addictiveness is its most dangerous quality. Fortunately, nicotine taken as gum or from the patch does not have the same power as nicotine taken as smoke. Most of the more dangerous effects of cigarettes come from inhaling the smoke, not simply from exposure to the nicotine. The gum and the patch are much safer than smoking.

History

The idea of helping smokers to quit by replacing the nicotine from their cigarettes with nicotine from another source is not entirely new. In the early 1940s, a scientist reported the effects of injecting nicotine directly into the bloodstream. This method, however, was impractical to help smokers. It was not until much later that a new strategy to replace the nicotine source was introduced. In the early 1970s, investigators from Sweden reported the development of a gum that released nicotine slowly as it was chewed. It took ten more years, however, before it was available in the United States. Almost another ten years later, in 1992, another method of delivering nicotine, the nicotine patch, was approved in the United States.

Who Should and Who Shouldn't Use the Gum or Patch?

The gum and patch are designed for smokers who are physically dependent on nicotine. According to the manufacturer of Nicorette gum, the smokers most likely to benefit:

- smoke more than fifteen cigarettes per day.

- prefer brands of cigarettes with higher nicotine levels.

- usually inhale deeply and frequently.

- smoke their first cigarette within thirty minutes of rising in the morning.

- find the first cigarette in the morning to be one of the hardest to give up.

- smoke more frequently in the morning than the rest of the day.

- find it difficult to refrain from smoking in places where it is forbidden.

- smoke even when they are ill.

There are also people who should not use these products. The effects of nicotine on the heart are similar whether the exposure occurs through smoking or through the gum or patch. In either case, there is an increase in heart rate and blood pressure. For this reason, the nicotine gum and patch are not recommended for people who have recently had a heart attack, who have a history of potentially dangerous heart-rhythm disturbances, or who have significant coronary artery disease.

Also, a woman who is pregnant or trying to become pregnant should not use nicotine gum or the nicotine patch. Nicotine (whether the exposure is by smoking, gum, or patch) may harm the fetus, possibly by causing decreased blood flow to the uterus. Nicotine should also be avoided while a woman is breastfeeding since nicotine passes freely into breast milk.

Individuals with a history of inflammation either in the esophagus or farther down the intestinal tract, or who have stomach ulcers, should only use the gum with extreme caution. The same thing goes for those individuals who have inflammation in the mouth or throat.

It should be noted, however, that for all of these people, nicotine replacement with the patch or gum is probably safer than the continued use of cigarettes.

Nicotine Gum

The Nicorette brand of gum was introduced to the public in the spring of 1984. It was heavily promoted through a multimillion dollar marketing campaign. Consequently, it soon became one of the fastest selling prescription medications, with sales exceeding $50 million within its first three years. There are estimates that one-tenth of all smokers have used this product.

Description of the Product

Nicotine polacrilex chewing gum is a sugar-free gum that is distributed by Marion-Merrell Dow Pharmaceuticals under the brand name Nicorette (nicotine resin complex). It is available only by prescription. Each piece of regular-strength gum contains 2 milligrams of nicotine and each piece of double-strength Nicorette DS gum contains 4 milligrams. Both also contain other chemicals, such as antacids, which help the mouth membranes absorb the nicotine.

How It Works

When the sugar-free nicotine gum combines with saliva and the pressure of your teeth, the nicotine is slowly released. When the gum is used, the amount of nicotine in the blood rises slowly, but it never reaches the levels achieved by regular cigarette smoking. After twenty to thirty minutes of use, almost all the nicotine in the gum is absorbed through your mouth and delivered into your bloodstream. The exact level of nicotine varies from person to person and from use to use.

Effectiveness

There is little dispute that nicotine gum alleviates many of the withdrawal symptoms associated with smoking cessation. Many studies have confirmed this finding. It's interesting, though, that the gum does not seem to suppress all the symptoms equally. For example, irritability seems to be blunted or reduced, but the craving, or the strong urge to smoke, is not always decreased. Also, hunger, depression, anxiety, and many other symptoms are reduced in some smokers using the gum but not in others. There is some evidence that weight gain can be lessened by the gum.

However, the most important question about nicotine gum is whether or not the replacement helps smokers quit. Although several studies have investigated this question, there remains some controversy about the gum's effectiveness. One of the problems is that there really isn't any conclusive research that shows whether or not smokers stay off tobacco once they stop using the nicotine gum. Don't be surprised if you hear different points of view about this popular intervention.

Nevertheless, most authorities believe that nicotine gum can be an effective aid to smoking cessation. After years of research, two factors have emerged as important to the success of nicotine gum. First, it must be given in an adequate dosage. This means that you must use it as prescribed (more about this below). Second, the gum must be accompanied by a structured quit-smoking program. This is a fairly surprising finding that has been confirmed by many studies. They show that if prescribed nicotine gum is used without any other quit-smoking strategies, it does little to increase the success rates of smokers trying to quit. The explanation is that the gum helps physical dependence but does nothing for psychological dependence.

Proper Use of the Gum

First, you must stop smoking. The gum is neither safe nor effective if used while you are smoking. The gum should *not* be used to help you cut down. It should only be used once you have quit. Why? One of the important benefits of the gum is that, unlike a cigarette, it does not produce a sudden high level of nicotine. This lower level of nicotine is what helps you decrease your dependence on the drug. Unfortunately, this benefit is erased if you smoke. Remember: It is *not* a tool to help you *cut down* on cigarettes. Further, this gum should *not* be chewed like regular gum. It is a medication.

Chewing Procedure

Nicotine is absorbed through your gums. Therefore, moisten the gum and bite down on it slowly. You should feel a peppery taste or tingling when the nicotine is released. When you notice this feeling, "park" the gum between your cheek and gums. When the feeling goes away, probably in about a minute, chew again until it returns. Repeat the process. (Don't worry if you swallow the gum. You should not feel any side effects.)

The reason for the starting-and-stopping chewing pattern is to get the maximum nicotine benefit without getting sick. Each piece should be used for twenty to thirty minutes and then discarded. It may take up to twenty minutes for nicotine from the gum to be absorbed by your body. Therefore, try to anticipate your cravings for a cigarette, from which the nicotine takes only seven seconds to get into your body! If too much time goes by between the start of your craving for a cigarette and when you take the gum, your resolve as an ex-smoker may weaken. You want the gum to help you remain an ex-smoker, right?

Common Misconception

Some people feel that you should quickly swallow the juices from the gum because, they believe, this is the way the nicotine is absorbed. This is simply not true. The truth is that nicotine absorbed from the stomach is quickly deactivated by the liver.

How Much Gum Should You Use?

The gum should be used liberally to prevent or treat withdrawal symptoms. Furthermore, the gum should be used for at least a few months. In the first month, do not worry about the amount you chew as long as it is under thirty pieces a day. Although its use is not officially recommended for longer than six months, some people use it for much longer. If you do discontinue use of the gum, you may want to carry some with you anyway, in case a craving hits.

With the recent FDA approval of the high-dose formulation of gum, Nicorette DS, which has 4 milligrams of nicotine as compared to the regular-strength gum's 2 milligrams, it is now possible to design a gum program in which you taper your exposure to nicotine over a period of a few months. Smokers who are heavily dependent on nicotine can begin their smoking-cessation program with the high-dose gum, then can move down to the low-dose gum.

Warning

Coffee, juices, and carbonated beverages block the absorption of nicotine from the gum. It seems that these beverages change the chemistry of saliva just enough to make nicotine gum ineffective. This was discovered by some researchers who noticed that many chewers did not receive the dose of nicotine that they expected they would. Many of these people drank coffee, fruit juices, or soft drinks either just before or while chewing the gum. A careful experiment proved the researchers' suspicions to be true. The current recommendation, therefore, is to avoid these drinks just before or while the gum is chewed.

Stopping the Gum

Despite the recommendation that nicotine gum not be used for more than a few months, many people find it difficult to stop. It seems that about one in twenty smokers who turn to the gum still chew it one year later. Of the smokers who are successful in quitting cigarettes with the use of nicotine gum, one in four continues using the gum up to one year later.

Long-term use is not known to cause health problems. The gum is what many people believe is keeping them free of cigarettes. Given that the gum does not contain the tar, carbon monoxide, and other harmful components of smoke, it seems preferable to smoking. In this way, it seems, the gum is helping both the physiological and psychological dependence.

When you are ready, give up the gum gradually. Since the gum does contain nicotine, if you stop abruptly you may feel some physical withdrawal. Most people find the process mostly painless.

Side Effects

There are some side effects associated with nicotine gum, but they occur rarely and are often minor, relating either to the gum chewing itself or to the chemical. They include problems with dental work, aching jaw muscles, mouth irritation, excessive salivation, indigestion, dizziness, insomnia, headaches, irritability, hiccups, lack of appetite, and, more commonly, abdominal discomfort, nausea, and indigestion.

Overdosage almost never occurs accidentally. Symptoms of acute nicotine overdose include nausea, salivation, abdominal pain, vomiting, diarrhea, cold sweats, headache, dizziness, and confusion.

Getting the Gum

Nicotine gum must be prescribed by a physician. However, any physician who merely writes you a prescription for the gum is not really helping you. The prescription should be accompanied by a plan to quit smoking, preferably one that is organized and structured. You should also be instructed on the use of the gum.

Nicotine Patch

Nicotine patches were introduced in 1992 amid much fanfare. Millions of dollars have been spent advertising the merits of this smoking-cessation method. Newspapers and magazines are sprinkled with ads promoting the patch. Fortunately, this is a case in which the product will likely live up to its billing!

Description

Most nicotine patches look like large round Band-Aids. They contain a small amount of nicotine embedded in a special material. This material is kept in close contact with the skin by an adhesive.

How It Works

The patch releases nicotine, which is absorbed by the skin. The nicotine then enters the bloodstream. The amount of nicotine absorbed from the patch is lower than that provided by smoking a cigarette.

It has been known for a while that nicotine can penetrate intact skin. Over the last decade, a few investigators have studied nicotine patches and found that skin absorption of nicotine could decrease cigarette cravings. Soon thereafter a patch was developed that could release small amounts of nicotine over a twenty-four-hour period.

Effectiveness

There are many reports that the nicotine patch reduces cigarette cravings, and recent findings have demonstrated that it can improve success rates among smokers who want to quit.

A recent report in *The New England Journal of Medicine* studied the safety and effectiveness of nicotine skin patches designed to release nicotine into the smoker's body over a sixteen-hour period. Subjects were given patches that were to be placed on the skin in the morning and taken off at night. Some were given patches that did not contain nicotine. No special counseling program accompanied this intervention.

The researchers found that the subjects given the real nicotine patches were more successful in quitting. The success rate at six weeks was 53 percent in the nicotine-patch group and 17 percent in the other. At the end of a year, the success rate was 17 percent in the nicotine-patch group and 4 percent in the other group. Symptoms of nicotine withdrawal tended to be less in the nicotine-patch group.

Another study involved nine medical centers and 935 patients. At the six-month mark, 1 in 4 subjects treated with the nicotine patch remained a nonsmoker as compared with 1 in 9 subjects treated with a patch that contained no nicotine.

These studies provide compelling scientific evidence that the patch is an effective aid for smoking cessation. There are few other methods that have undergone such screening by the medical community and have been found to be beneficial.

How to Use the Patch

The patches come in various strengths including 22, 21, 15, 14, 11, 10, 7, and 5 milligrams, depending on the manufacturer. The size of the patch is proportional to the amount of nicotine in it. Therefore, the 21-milligram patch is the largest and the 7-milligram patch is the smallest.

The patches may be used in a variety of different programs. One approach is to use a larger patch for six weeks and then move to smaller patches for two weeks each. Some people use the larger patch for a longer time. There is no magic way to tell when you are ready to switch to a smaller patch.

It is usually recommended that at six weeks you give a smaller patch a try. If you have trouble with symptoms when you switch, then you can always return to the larger patch. As with the nicotine gum, you should *not* use the patch unless you have stopped smoking.

The importance of this warning is highlighted by the recent reports of heart attacks in people who were wearing a patch and smoking. Although the contribution of the double dose of nicotine to the heart attack cannot be proven, there is concern among some physicians that the added nicotine played a role.

How to Place the Patch

The patch is designed to be placed on any nonhairy, clean, dry area of the body. The exact location of the patch does not matter. You should avoid areas that are oily, dirty, hairy, or irritated in any way. Open the storage packet and remove the patch. Place the patch on your skin and hold it there for about ten seconds, until you are sure that it sticks well. The entire patch, including the edges, should be firmly attached. Once you have placed the patch, you should wash your hands, since if you get nicotine in your eyes or nose, it could cause burning, stinging, or redness. The patch should remain in place for twenty-four hours and then be discarded. (Discard the patches in a place that is safe from children and pets.) If you leave the patch on for longer than twenty-four hours, it can irritate your skin. The next patch should be placed in a different location. You should not use one particular skin location more than once a week.

Side Effects

In recent large studies of the nicotine patch, there have been very few reported side effects. The most common complaint has been mild itchiness that lasted for fifteen to thirty minutes after placing the patch on the skin.

Common Questions About the Nicotine Patch

Does it matter at what time of day you apply the patch?

The time of day is not important. The patch can be put on at any time of the day or night, and this time can vary. All that you need to do is take off the old one and put on the new one.

What if you leave the patch on for longer than twenty-four hours?

Don't worry. The recommendation that the patch not be worn for longer than twenty-four hours is based on the observation that it may cause skin irritation. There should not be any other ill effects. Just remove the patch when you can.

Can you take a shower if you're wearing the patch?

The patch was designed to get wet without losing adhesiveness or effectiveness. You can bathe, swim, or shower while wearing it.

What if the patch falls off?

The patch is designed to stick well. If it does fall off, however, simply replace it. It is a good idea to carry an extra patch with you just in case you need it.

Which patch should you use?

Four nicotine-releasing adhesive patches for the skin—Nicoderm, Habitrol, Prostep, and Nicotrol—have been approved for the relief of nicotine withdrawal symptoms. They are all excellent products. Nicoderm and Habitrol are available in strengths of 7, 14, and 21 milligrams per day. Prostep is available in 11 and 22 milligrams per day, and Nicotrol is available in 5, 10, and 15 milligrams per day.

Nicotrol is designed to be worn only during waking hours, while the other patches should be worn for twenty-four hours. Nicotrol claims this is an advantage, but there is no evidence that indicates this patch is better than the others. In fact, there are no published comparisons of these patches in any clinical trials. Nevertheless, there are claims by the pharmaceutical companies that there are important differences in these patches relating to blood levels of nicotine, rate of allergic reactions, and ease of opening the package. At this time, all of the patches should be considered equally effective. The prices are similar; they average three dollars a day. The bottom line is that they are all excellent products and there is currently no clear advantage to using one over the others.

Which dose should you use?

Patches should usually be started at the strongest strength. For Nicoderm and Habitrol, you should start with 21 milligrams per day; for Prostep, the 22-milligram strength; and for Nicotrol, 15 milligrams. For smokers who weigh less than 100 pounds, smoke less than half a pack of cigarettes per day, or who have cardiovascular disease, it may be preferable to start with a lower dose.

Physicians and Nicotine Replacement

Physicians may not always be the best source of information about nicotine replacement. A recent survey of California physicians practicing general medicine revealed that many were misinformed about the use of nicotine gum, even though almost 90 percent had prescribed it within the last year. Almost half of these physicians believed that, even if their patients did not stop smoking, they should use the gum to cut down on cigarettes. In addition, contrary to recommendations from authorities on smoking cessation, one in four of the doctors thought that the gum should not be used for more than one month.

The message is that not all doctors are informed (or even interested) in smoking cessation. It is your responsibility to educate yourself. If you are ready to quit, find a physician who knows about the gum or is familiar with the patch and has experience prescribing it.

Should You Use the Gum or the Patch?

In many ways, the patch may be an improvement over the gum. The use of the patch is easy to master. It is unobtrusive and socially acceptable. Also, it may be better for you to be exposed to a low level of nicotine over sixteen or twenty-four hours rather than to the small bursts that the gum provides. No one has yet, however, compared the gum to the patch. Since the gum has been in use for almost ten years in this country, it remains an important standard strategy. It can also satisfy the need of some smokers for oral stimulation. The important point is that nicotine replacement, whether by gum or patch, is one of the best methods of helping you to quit smoking. Its benefit is proven scientifically by studies published in prestigious medical journals.

Recommendation

The cost of the gum or the patch seems well worth the investment. If you feel that you are dependent on nicotine, you should determine if your physician is familiar with these methods and consider using either the gum or the patch to help you quit. If you use these methods, however, you should combine them with an organized program for the best results.

POSSIBILITIES FOR FUTURE NICOTINE SUBSTITUTION

While nicotine gum is being widely used and the nicotine patch is the current rage, other methods of administering nicotine are being developed. Among those that scientists are currently testing are nicotine nasal sprays, smokeless cigarettes, and nicotine aerosols.

Nicotine nasal spray administers nicotine via gel-like droplets of liquid. Patients can achieve higher levels of nicotine with the spray than with the gum. Each pump of the spray bottle delivers about one-half milligram of nicotine, and repeated pumps can give you exposure to the same amount of nicotine as in a cigarette.

Some researchers are very optimistic about the nasal spray. In the August 8, 1988, issue of the British medical journal *The Lancet*, a group of researchers from London confirmed that nasal nicotine spray is truly effective as an aid to smoking cessation. The group studied the value of the nasal spray in over 200 smokers by giving real nicotine spray to half of the subjects and spray that did not contain nicotine to the other half. The subjects were not told which spray they had. Both groups attended quit-smoking sessions designed to help them succeed. After one year, the group that used the nasal spray with nicotine was more than twice as likely to be successful than the nicotine-less group (26 percent versus 10 percent). The benefit of the nicotine spray was greatest for the heaviest smokers. The spray reduced withdrawal symptoms, cravings, and weight gain. There were no serious side effects reported, although some people found the spray irritating at first. The biggest problem may be that many people are too embarrassed to squirt liquid into their nose in public. Advocates of the spray claim that it may be better than the gum or patch because, like cigarettes, it provides a burst of exposure to nicotine. There is, however, no evidence that it is better than what is already available.

A smokeless cigarette is also being investigated. This is a plastic, cigarette-shaped tube. It contains a nicotine-soaked fibrous material that provides a dose of nicotine each time it's dragged on. Since it is not lit, its use can be extended way beyond that of a cigarette.

In addition, a nicotine aerosol is being developed. This device allows nicotine to be inhaled without cigarette smoke. It may be helpful for people who need a boost of nicotine greater than what the gum or nasal spray can provide.

WARNING

Nicotine replacement does not guarantee success in your quest to quit smoking. It can help you, but the responsibility for success remains yours. Do not be lulled into thinking that this method will accomplish this challenging task for you.

CHAPTER 6

The Smoking-Reduction Strategy

Weaning Yourself From Cigarettes

Some smokers cannot face the idea of quitting cigarettes cold turkey. Those who don't try nicotine replacement may prefer to gradually wean themselves, either by cutting down by degrees through the use of special filters or by switching to cigarettes with lower tar and nicotine ratings. This section reviews the relative merits of these "controlled smoking" strategies.

SWITCHING DOWN BRANDS: NICOTINE FADING

Let's talk about a technique called nicotine fading. This involves switching to brands of cigarettes with progressively lower amounts of tar and nicotine until (hopefully) you're finally able to quit.

What is the idea behind this? Gradually reducing the amount of nicotine you consume may ease the process of quitting. And there's another train of thought behind this technique: smokers who are unable to quit completely think that they are better off switching to a brand with a lower tar and nicotine rating. Unfortunately, individuals using this procedure tend to smoke more, smoke each cigarette longer, and are unhappy with the smoking process; yet, they continue it.

This strategy is currently used only in a few treatment programs. But the idea that it is good to switch to a brand with a low tar and nicotine rating is a popular belief that is reinforced by attractive ads for low-tar and low-nicotine cigarettes. Many smokers use low-yield cigarettes as a transition to quitting, even if they have never heard of the technique called nicotine fading. Physicians have even recommended that smokers who are unable, or unwilling, to quit switch to low-yield cigarettes for "health reasons."

What Is the Truth?

Low-tar and low-nicotine cigarettes are a trap for smokers. Advertisements make them seem like a great idea. They suggest that you can still smoke and lower your exposure to tar and nicotine. In the fight for market share, low-yield alternatives to the popular higher tar and nicotine brands such as Winston, Camel, and Marlboro portray themselves as the "healthy choice." They seem to say, "If you must smoke, smoke us."

Unfortunately, the truth is that low-tar and low-nicotine cigarettes do not reduce your exposure to tar and nicotine. You are no better off smoking these cigarettes than any other brand. In fact, studies of the effect of low-yield cigarettes have found no relationship between a cigarette's published yield and a smoker's intake of nicotine, as measured by a blood test. A study published in 1983 in *The New England Journal of Medicine* concluded that smokers of low-nicotine cigarettes do not consume less nicotine.

Many other studies support these results. In addition, experts have stated that the increased risk of heart attacks is no different for smokers of high-yield cigarettes than it is for smokers of low-yield cigarettes. Other investigators have reported that levels of carbon monoxide in the blood are no different either.

How is it possible that these low-tar and low-nicotine cigarettes are not what they say? Let's discuss how these cigarettes are produced. Low-yield cigarettes do not contain any special, different kind of tobacco. The tobacco in these cigarettes has the same amount and concentration of nicotine as any other brand. So what's the so-called advantage? The "benefit" is achieved by using filters that mix the inhaled smoke with some air. In addition, the tobacco burns more rapidly. These advantages, however, do not translate into lower exposure for the smoker. Remember: you do *not* help yourself by smoking these cigarettes. Are you confused? This whole topic is confusing. Let's try to clear it up.

The Weaknesses of Tar and Nicotine Measurement

The United States Federal Trade Commission (FTC) determines tar and nicotine yields of cigarettes by using smoking machines. These machines draw short puffs with a small syringe at pre-set times until a certain length of cigarette is burned. The smoke collected is then analyzed for tar and nicotine content. If the cigarette burns quickly, the machine takes fewer puffs by the time the proper length is reached. Fewer puffs result in less tar and nicotine being collected.

In addition, manufacturers have developed filters that mix the smoke with air. This further reduces the tar and nicotine measured by the machine. This mixing, also called ventilation, is usually accomplished by placing small holes in the filter. Yes, these techniques do work well to reduce the machine's collection of tar and nicotine. But, unfortunately, despite all the hype, there is still no evidence that these cigarettes reduce your exposure to tar and nicotine.

If you're uncomfortable with a filter, you'll vary the depth of your puffs. In addition, you'll vary the number of puffs you take with each cigarette. After all, you're not consciously thinking about this as you smoke, are you? Some smokers even unwittingly circumvent the filter by holding the cigarette in such a way that the holes are covered. And you may have seen some smokers tear off the filters on some cigarettes.

The message is clear. Switching to low-tar and low-nicotine cigarettes does not reduce your exposure to cigarette smoke or your risk of developing diseases associated with smoking. Therefore, smoking these cigarettes is not a reasonable alternative to quitting. Switching to brands with lower ratings before you quit probably does little to wean you off nicotine. There are over twenty medical studies on nicotine fading. Most found no important benefits. It is widely felt that smokers compensate by consuming about the same nicotine no matter what brand they smoke. With all of this information, it is difficult to justify nicotine fading as a contribution to the quitting process.

There is only one possible benefit, and it is a psychological one. If you use this technique, you may feel that you're making progress as you make each brand switch. This may provide you with the necessary confidence that will lead to your quitting. But if you don't follow through and quit completely, it would be wrong to assume that you're improving your health simply because you're now smoking low-yield cigarettes.

FILTERS

You can obtain a variety of smoking filters at local drug stores. These filters are being marketed as another way to help smokers gradually wean themselves off nicotine. These products often come as a set that is supposed to filter progressively more nicotine from the smoke you inhale. It's usually suggested that they be used over a four- to eight-week period. Some of the filters are designed to be reusable, whereas others can be thrown away. There are remarkably few studies of these filters in medical literature.

One recent entry in this market is a product called Kick the Habit, which is sold as a gradual smoking-withdrawal system. It is touted as working better than brand switching. (This claim is less impressive when you realize that brand switching is not very effective!)

The Kick the Habit product contains cards and pamphlets to increase your motivation. The main component, though, is a set of graduated filters designed to remove 25 percent, then 50 percent, and then 75 percent of the nicotine you would inhale. There are enough filters in each set to last three weeks.

Viadent, the company that produces Kick the Habit, says that it does not have any information on quit-rates because the product is so new. A very preliminary study from the University of Minnesota suggests that these filters produce significant reductions in nicotine exposure. However, the study was unable to show that the filters help smokers to quit successfully. It recommends more studies. So far none of the major medical journals have published an article showing that this method is effective.

At this point, there is only suggestive evidence to support the use of graduated filters. More studies need to be done before products like Kick the Habit can be fully recommended. Nevertheless, these products are simple, nontoxic, and relatively inexpensive (about thirty dollars). They can't hurt you, they may reduce the amount of tar and nicotine you inhale, and they may be helpful to some smokers.

Although these products may sound like they make sense, critics say that smokers will simply drag more deeply and smoke more often to compensate. Other products loosely in this category punch holes into a cigarette's existing filter, hoping to gradually reduce the amount of tar and nicotine you inhale. This is because the holes in the filter introduce more air in the smoke, thereby diluting it. This is similar to the method used in low-yield cigarettes mentioned earlier. And we know how beneficial *that* is.

GRADUAL REDUCTION (TAPERING)

Many people who are long-term smokers prefer the idea of stopping gradually because they feel it would be easier. If it works, why not? Because researchers have suggested that rarely does gradual reduction result in long-term elimination of the smoking habit. In fact, smokers who have tried to cut down gradually have, in a number of studies, experienced cigarette cravings as strong as those of smokers who stopped cold turkey. Another negative: the cravings soon pass if you stop all at once. But if you try to stop by gradual reduction and the cravings continue, what good is it?

If you are insistent that gradual reduction is the only way you can quit, we won't tell you not to. After all, we do want you to be successful. So here are a number of guidelines to try to incorporate in your tapering program:

- Try not to smoke automatically. Put your cigarettes, lighters, ashtrays, and other smoking paraphernalia in a place that will require effort to reach when you decide to smoke.

- Only smoke the cigarettes you really want. Yes, ask yourself the question, "Do I really want it?" before lighting up.

- Try to smoke less and less of each cigarette. You might want to draw a line on it, indicating where you'll stop. Make sure you put it out when you reach the spot.

- After you get a craving, try postponing lighting up for longer and longer periods of time.

- Smoke under adverse, unpleasant conditions (such as out in the cold, standing up, or before a meal).

- Smoke a brand of cigarettes you dislike.

- Don't buy large quantities of cigarettes. Try to buy only one pack at a time, making it harder for you to get them.

- Predetermine when, where, and why you'll smoke. Also predetermine how many cigarettes you'll smoke in a day.

There are many other guidelines you can incorporate. Of course, they're *not* designed to make smoking pleasant. They're intended to remind you more and more frequently of how ludicrous the whole process of smoking is (besides being unhealthy) so you'll finally just fling your arms up in the air (along with your cigarette!) and say, "Enough. I quit!"

But no matter which method you use or which guidelines you follow, there are several important things you should focus on. You should always:

- Decrease the number of puffs you take from each cigarette.

- Decrease the depth you inhale each puff.

- Decrease the length of each drag.

- Increase the time between puffs.

- Increase the time between cigarettes.

These are the basics.

GADGETS

There are also gadgets designed to help you gradually reduce your dependence on cigarettes and eventually quit. Despite their hype, however, they are just variations on the same theme.

For example, one popular new product is a palm-size computer called Life Sign. The computer records your smoking habits, develops a personalized program to quit, and guides you through it. This is how it works: For seven days you record each cigarette that you smoke by pushing a button on the computer. The computer remembers when you smoke and develops a personalized profile of your smoking habit. It then constructs a withdrawal program for you that lasts from two to five weeks, depending on how many cigarettes you usually smoke. The computer displays the number of days until your quit date and tells you when you can smoke your next cigarette. The idea is to disrupt your ordinary smoking pattern and have you smoke at random times. This strategy is supposed to separate the act of smoking from the cues that cause the urge to smoke. Gradually, the time between cigarettes is lengthened. The goal is to assist you in achieving total abstinence from cigarettes. The computer even makes allowances for slips. For example, if you slip with an unscheduled cigarette (and push a button on the computer), it will adjust your program.

This product is not cheap. It runs about eighty dollars for the computer, an instruction manual, and, in some cases, an instructional video. There is a discount program if the product is ordered in quantity.

Is there evidence to support this program? The company claims that the product has been studied scientifically, but there are no articles substantiating this in any major medical journal. There are, however, a few brief reports about the product, but it is not clear how it compares to other quit-smoking techniques.

So, despite the claims of the manufacturer that the product is "successful, cost-effective, and easy to use," there is no proof that it is anything more than easy to use. However, the idea is attractive and may appeal to some smokers. It has been reported that more than 600,000 of these units have been sold since it was introduced in 1991.

Our major concern is the cost of this unproven method. It may be worth a try, but when you cut through the hype, you'll realize that this technique has not yet been embraced by the scientific community. Even if it helps you to quit, it is not certain that it aids you in steering clear of cigarettes later.

Another gadget designed to help you gradually reduce your cigarette consumption is Smoke and Stop, a cigarette case with a timer lock. You set the case to open at preset intervals, thereby controlling your access to cigarettes. Over time, you gradually increase the period between openings. There are no studies on the effectiveness of this product in mainstream medical literature. However, it's hard to believe that a locked cigarette case would stymie someone who really wanted a cigarette. At a cost of about eighty dollars, it's hard to justify its use.

As we mentioned, gradually reducing the number of cigarettes you smoke is a common way to attempt to quit. Unfortunately, despite the few success stories you may occasionally hear, tapering rarely works. By extending the quitting process, it becomes extremely difficult to give up those final few cigarettes. Further, virtually any physical or psychological trigger can increase the number of cigarettes smoked to the previous high level (if not higher!).

Smokers who try tapering feel a constant sense of deprivation. They often find it almost impossible to sustain their effort to achieve success. Yes, some people have done it, and some programs encourage it. The hope is that, if you reduce to just a few cigarettes, you'll come to your senses, realize what a horrible habit smoking is, and just stop from that point. A small percentage of individuals has stopped smoking for this reason. But, in general, you already *have* come to your senses. You do realize what a horrible habit it is (or you're learning!). So why not just stop?

Why do some people like the idea of tapering? Well, the prospect of "here one day, gone the next" (about your cigarettes, of course!) may be terrifying. You may feel this is the only way to really psyche yourself to get past this panic.

In all probability, the only real advantage of tapering is that it can remind you of your commitment to a program of giving up smoking. But once you're fully aware of this commitment, and you can use other much more effective techniques to stop and get it over with, which makes more sense?

CHAPTER 7
The Medication Strategy
Using Prescription Drugs

Since the beginning of this century, people have touted elixirs, tablets, mouthwashes, and teas containing special ingredients as ways to help smokers escape from the urge to smoke. While some of these products are truly designed to help smokers, others take advantage of the public's trust.

Smokers are particularly susceptible to claims that a medication can help them quit, since most of them know how difficult it is. Many are desperate for a way to make the process easier. The idea that simply taking a medication can help you beat the craving for cigarettes is extremely attractive.

There are many medications that are touted for their ability to help you quit. Yes, some of them may be helpful, but others are almost certainly not. In some cases, certain medications can actually harm you.

Remember that any product should be proven as useful before it is recommended. Don't consider any medication to be effective until it is verified as such. In some cases, you may hear contradictory comments about the same medication. If that's so, whether or not you buy it depends on your instincts. Remember that practically every medication has side effects and that, despite the hype, no medication will accomplish your goal in place of your efforts. There is no special medication that will quit smoking for you.

This section reviews various medications that are prescribed or marketed for smokers. It focuses on clonidine, antidepressant medications, sedatives, and mecamylamine. Other medications, like nicotine, lobeline, and silver acetate, are discussed in other chapters.

CLONIDINE

Clonidine is a medication that is currently used to treat high blood pressure. It has received attention in the popular press because it has also been used to treat nicotine withdrawal symptoms.

Preparation

Clonidine is a prescription medication that can be used only under a physician's supervision. It is available as pills or as a patch that is placed on the skin weekly. For smoking cessation, clonidine is usually prescribed at approximately .15 to .2 milligrams per day or in a patch that provides an equivalent dosage.

History

Clonidine was developed in the late 1960s as a nasal decongestant. It became a blood pressure medicine after it was observed to lower blood pressure as a side effect during its early tests.

In the late 1970s, it was also learned that clonidine seemed to help drug addicts who were withdrawing. Some authorities believe that clonidine is as effective as methadone, and a few facilities use it in their drug withdrawal programs. Alcohol withdrawal programs have also used clonidine with some limited success.

With the growing realization that smoking is an addiction, it was only natural that someone would try clonidine for nicotine withdrawal. In 1984, in the journal *Science*, investigators from Columbia University reported that clonidine reduced the craving for cigarettes during the first day after quitting. This study generated hope that clonidine would be the answer to nicotine withdrawal symptoms. But subsequent studies have had difficulty proving whether clonidine can reliably help a smoker quit.

How It Works

A lot of medical information is available about clonidine's ability to activate certain parts of the brain, but very little is understood about how it affects blood pressure or blunts withdrawal symptoms.

Effectiveness

There is some controversy about the effectiveness of clonidine. One study of almost 200 smokers found that the drug made no difference in smoking-cessation success rates after the first week. Another study, however, did find that the success rate in smokers treated with clonidine was twice that of the group that wasn't treated.

The difficulty in proving the value of clonidine is highlighted by a recent study from Rochester, New York. Smokers were recruited from among patients visiting their physicians for routine health care. Smokers who agreed to participate were given pills to take each day. Half the smokers received clonidine pills and half received a placebo, a pill without any active medication. Neither the smokers nor their physicians knew whether they had taken clonidine. All subjects were asked to report their withdrawal symptoms. Surprisingly, the group taking the placebo had fewer symptoms! After four weeks, there were no differences in the success rates of the two groups.

This study seems to strongly suggest that clonidine is not helpful. After presenting their results, however, the authors of this report admitted that their study could not absolutely conclude that clonidine was useless. They suggested that a truly definitive study would require over 24,000 participants and is unlikely ever to be performed. Therefore, there will probably continue to be some uncertainty about the benefits of clonidine on smoking cessation. Currently, clonidine is not officially approved by the FDA for this purpose. Therefore, the company that produces clonidine is not actively marketing it for smoking cessation.

Side Effects

The major side effects of clonidine are dry mouth, drowsiness, and constipation. Many other less common side effects have also been reported.

The danger of clonidine is that if it is stopped suddenly after prolonged use, it may cause very high blood pressure. In addition, abrupt discontinuation of the medicine may cause nervousness and anxiety as well as flushing, nausea, and vomiting. These reactions can usually be avoided if the dosage is reduced gradually, over two to four days.

Recommendation

Clonidine should not be your first choice for your personalized program. As nice as it would be to have a magic pill that makes it easy to quit smoking, clonidine does not seem to be it. There is no definite evidence to support its use. Nevertheless, if you have failed at other attempts and want to try a new method, no one can tell you that clonidine is useless. In addition, used under a physician's direction, it is unlikely to be harmful. Consequently, it falls into the "perhaps worth a try" category.

DOXEPIN

Doxepin is an antidepressant medication. Recently, it has been tried as an aid to smoking cessation.

Preparation

Doxepin pills are available by prescription. In most recent studies, this is how doxepin was prescribed for smoking cessation: 50 milligrams taken before bedtime on the first three days, 100 milligrams taken before bedtime on days four through six, and 150 milligrams taken before bedtime on days seven through forty-nine. Then the medication was stopped.

History

In the 1940s, two scientists developed a group of substances to help treat the common cold. Instead of finding the perfect cold remedy, they discovered that one of the chemical compounds that they examined had a calming effect. With more research it was found that this medicine, imipramine, had a remarkable ability to improve the mood of depressed patients. Subsequently, a class of medications, called tricyclic antidepressants, was developed.

Doctors have used tricyclic antidepressants to treat depression for years. The use of these medications, especially doxepin (the trade names are Adavin and Sinequan), as an aid to smoking cessation is much more recent. Some scientists noted that certain nicotine withdrawal symptoms were similar to those of depression. This observation may have led to the idea of trying tricyclic antidepressant agents.

These medications are considered potentially useful for many people who are trying to quit. There appears to be a strong association between cigarette smoking and depression. A recent study showed that smokers are more likely than nonsmokers to have a problem with depression at some time in their life. In addition, smokers who have a history of depression tend to have a lower success rate when they attempt to quit. This may be another reason to watch for symptoms of depression (depressed mood, diminished interest in most activities, weight loss or weight gain, sleepiness or insomnia, feelings of worthlessness, difficulty concentrating, recurring thoughts of dying or suicide) and be treated promptly.

Effectiveness

There are very few studies of the effectiveness of doxepin. One of the first, published in 1989, found that individuals given doxepin had less frequent and less severe withdrawal symptoms than individuals given a placebo. Unfortunately, the patients on doxepin were not significantly more successful in quitting. However, another study did find some benefits to taking doxepin.

Medical literature also contains a few scattered reports that investigate other antidepressant agents. These studies have used very small numbers of people. Therefore, it is difficult to make conclusions about these medications. Currently, no tricyclic antidepressant is approved by the FDA as an aid to smoking cessation.

Side Effects

The biggest problem with tricyclic antidepressants is that they can have unpleasant side effects. The drugs can cause dry mouth, constipation, a sour taste, dizziness, upset stomach, palpitations, and difficulty urinating. These symptoms do not happen to everyone, but they are common.

Recommendation

More studies of antidepressants are needed. These drugs should not become an aid to quitting unless their benefit can be shown more persuasively. Nevertheless, they may eventually play an important role in helping smokers.

However, if you think that you are depressed, be sure to be evaluated by a professional. This not only may help you in your smoking cessation effort, but can also help you improve your overall quality of life. Our concerns about the drugs reflect our uncertainty about their ability to help you quit smoking and do not relate to their effectiveness as antidepressant agents.

OTHER MEDICATIONS

From time to time, a variety of medications has been mentioned as agents to facilitate smoking cessation. None are approved by the FDA for this purpose. However, mecamylamine and sedatives deserve mention.

Mecamylamine takes a slightly different approach from the medications that are designed to ease withdrawal symptoms. It blocks the effect of nicotine. Mecamylamine is designed to deny you the benefits of smoking.

Mecamylamine was originally marketed by Merck, Sharp and Dohme as an antihypertensive medication known as Inversine. It was introduced in the mid-1950s for the treatment of high blood pressure. There have been a few studies published that suggest that mecamylamine can decrease a smoker's desire for cigarettes and also lessen the satisfaction produced by smoking. However, the drug has never been widely used and there are no large studies that show it helps in quitting. Therefore, it cannot be recommended at this time.

Sedatives, like Valium and Xanax, are among the most commonly prescribed drugs in this country. They are often given to relax muscles, reduce anxiety, and treat insomnia. Unfortunately, some people become dependent on these medications, even after taking them as directed by their physician.

Sedatives should have no place in anyone's smoking-cessation program. They are neither approved nor recommended as an aid to quit smoking. There is no controversy in this area. No legitimate study has suggested that sedatives are effective in helping smokers to quit. Furthermore, these drugs can easily be abused and lead to dependence, even when used as prescribed by a physician. Given that these drugs are powerful, dangerous, and not effective, there is no reason that they should be used as an aid to quit smoking.

Why are we mentioning this class of drugs? In a recent survey of physicians who treat patients trying to quit smoking, more than one in four reported that they had prescribed sedatives during the previous year to help smokers quit smoking despite the lack of support for use of these drugs in smoking-cessation programs. Sedatives are often an easy choice for anxious patients who want to quit, but they are never the right choice.

Other medications mentioned for smoking cessation over the years are amphetamines, meprobamate, tranquilizers, and anti-epilepsy drugs. Again, none has emerged as clearly beneficial and all should be avoided as aids to quitting cigarettes.

CHAPTER 8
The Substitution Strategy
Finding Something New

Quitting cigarettes may make you feel that something is being taken away from you. Your body may feel the absence of nicotine. Your hands may fidget without the feel of a cigarette. Your mouth may miss the oral stimulation. Your image of yourself may feel incomplete without smoking. And physiologically, you may feel like you're having a harder time coping without cigarettes. Any of these feelings may be obstacles to your success.

One approach to dealing with your resistance to giving up cigarettes is to substitute something for them. The substitute may occupy your hands or mouth, replace the sensation in your airway, or divert your attention and energy altogether. This section reviews methods of replacing cigarettes, other than those covered in the nicotine-replacement section.

CHEWING GUM

Many smokers enjoy the oral stimulation of smoking. Chewing-gum companies occasionally focus on this fact. Some of them market their product to help smokers cope during times when they cannot light up. A number of recent advertising campaigns have emphasized this point.

Chewing gum is one of the easiest things you can do to help you quit smoking. Unfortunately, there is little scientific evidence about whether it will help you or not. Nevertheless, it is not considered harmful, so you have nothing to lose if you want to try chewing gum.

FAKE CIGARETTES

Fake cigarettes, sold in many pharmacies, are plastic imitations designed to give you something to hold. Some of them contain a fragrance or a slight minty taste. One executive from a large drug-store chain remembers that his superiors laughed when he first suggested that they carry the product. Now, it is one of their best-selling smoking-cessation aids!

These fake cigarettes may help you if you often feel like you have to keep your hands busy. They also give you something to "puff" on when you crave a cigarette. The benefit of this product is not clear. The problem is that although the fake cigarettes keep your hands busy, they may also remind you of smoking. The best that can be said of this strategy is that the cigarettes are cheap and harmless.

CITRIC-ACID AEROSOL

Some smokers say that they enjoy the distinctive sensation of smoke. This desire is confirmed by reports that smokers do not derive as much satisfaction from nicotine delivered in ways other than smoke. Some experts believe that the respiratory sensation is an important component of smoker satisfaction.

This theory was first tested by some researchers at the University of California at Los Angeles. They numbed the airways of smokers with an anaesthetic, allowed them to smoke, and then inquired about their satisfaction. Blocking the sensation of smoke dramatically decreased the overall satisfaction of these smokers, although they were being exposed to the same amount of nicotine.

These researchers then wondered if they could find a safe substitute for the sensation of smoking that would help smokers quit. They developed a fine aerosol containing a mildly irritating but nontoxic solution of citric acid (a substance found in lemons and limes). Their research suggested that this spray simulated the sensation of cigarette smoke. Further studies showed that smokers rated the sensation of the aerosol similar to their brand of cigarettes or at least as good as a low-tar and low-nicotine cigarette. Their results suggest that the aerosol may be used by smokers trying to quit as a way of decreasing the craving for cigarettes.

Larger studies proving the benefit of a citric-acid aerosol have not yet been published in major medical journals. Therefore, the real value of this intervention remains speculative. The aerosol mist is not yet readily available. For now, this approach remains experimental, although it appears promising and may be available in the future.

EXERCISE AND DIET

Good health practices tend to go together. Substituting regular exercise and a healthy diet for cigarettes may be a powerful contributor to your success. As you pay more attention to good health practices, smoking becomes more incompatible with your lifestyle.

Exercise

Exercise can be an excellent substitute activity. It can aid your success in quitting by helping you focus on exercise and health instead of smoking and risk. You'll feel better when you exercise, but you'll have to breathe better to perform adequately. Increasing exercise, therefore, can go hand-in-hand with the improved breathing that results from eliminating smoking.

Although there are some exceptions, smokers are less likely than nonsmokers to engage in regular exercise. Many former smokers have found that exercise programs are a good and useful complement to their smoking-cessation program.

You may be surprised to find that physical activity is more pleasurable after you quit smoking. Your body will work better as it gets further away from the chronic exposure to nicotine and cigarette smoke. You'll feel the difference!

What types of exercise can be helpful? The possibilities are endless and include tennis, swimming, dancing, skiing, calisthenics, jogging, bicycling, racquetball, or whatever else you would enjoy.

Your exercise doesn't have to be vigorous. The important point is to increase your physical activity. Even a short walk during the day can provide you with health benefits. Some smokers use physical activity as a substitute for cigarettes. It can combat cravings and help reduce stress.

Exercise is also useful in dealing with the possibility of weight gain after smoking cessation. You may find it hard to decrease your food intake in the first few weeks after you quit. The best way to counteract this problem is to increase your activity.

However, if you are interested in undertaking a new, vigorous exercise program, you should consult your physician first. Exercise brings about many benefits, but you want to make sure that your program is sensible and safe.

When you do begin, make sure you get yourself in shape gradually. Even though you may start slowly, do exercise regularly. Plan on scheduling an exercise period at least three times a week, otherwise you really won't experience the benefits.

Diet

As part of an overall strategy to improve your health, you may want to direct your attention toward your diet. Many smokers who quit find that this is very important. Nutritional programs in this country are currently moving away from foods with a high fat content. Carbohydrates, like bread and potatoes, once thought of as foods to be avoided, are now recommended.

Here are a few good guidelines for dietary improvement to help you quit without gaining weight:

- Drink water before meals and throughout the day.

- Substitute low-fat foods like fruits and vegetables, skim milk, and low-fat cottage cheese for high-fat foods whenever possible.

- Broil, bake, or boil foods instead of frying them.

- Anticipate your need to snack, and plan your snacks in advance. Try to include foods like raw vegetables and unbuttered popcorn. Have foods on hand for nibbling that are good for filling you up but low in fat content. For instance, fruits, air-popped popcorn, and low-salt pretzels are good options. Bring your snacks with you wherever you go.

- Use sugarless gum and hard candy to blunt your urges to snack.

- Think before you eat. Do not eat as a reflex. Give yourself a chance to decide if you are really hungry or if you're eating for another, less appropriate reason.

There are plenty of good books to read about ways to improve your diet. Check them out in libraries or bookstores. But make sure you adopt a healthy, well-rounded nutritional program. You don't want to exchange one bad habit for another, do you?

NEW ACTIVITIES

Treat yourself. Doing something nice for yourself as a substitute for smoking is another good strategy. Is there an activity or hobby that you have wanted to start? You're in the process of making a difficult but important change in your life. Finding pleasurable activities to interest you may make the time pass more easily as you get through the first few weeks and beyond. And, of course, the money you save from not purchasing cigarettes can be put toward a new activity or hobby!

CHAPTER 9

The Alternative Strategies

Using Acupuncture and Hypnosis

Acupuncture and hypnosis are two techniques that are considered by some to fall outside the realm of modern medicine. However, they have received attention as alternative methods to smoking cessation. They are usually offered by private practitioners who have various types and degrees of training. The services are offered in many different settings. These techniques may be attractive to some smokers. But remember—the aware consumer is the smart consumer.

ACUPUNCTURE

Acupuncture is an ancient Chinese technique, in practice for thousands of years, that has been used to promote, restore, and maintain health. The technique is accepted widely in China as an important part of traditional medicine and is considered superior to many more modern forms.

Acupuncture has captured the imagination of many Americans who perceive it as a simple, nonmedical approach. Its use has extended to the treatment of addictions. As a result, some people have applied it to the field of smoking cessation.

Acupuncturists claim there are a number of benefits that smokers who are trying to quit can experience. They include a reduction in physiological cravings for nicotine as well as a reduction in the consequences of nicotine withdrawal (such as nervousness, irritability, craving for food, or depression). Acupuncture can be very relaxing, and many people report that they fall into a restful sleep immediately following the treatment.

Description

Acupuncture involves the use of hair-thin needles or surgical-steel staples. The use of staples, which are tiny (about one-sixteenth of an inch), is also called staple puncture. The needles or staples are placed under the skin in predetermined parts of the body.

There is some controversy about the sites at which the needles or staples should be placed for smoking cessation. One common site that is said to induce loss of desire to smoke is at the center of the bottom of the ear. Needles are also commonly placed in both ears. In one program, the needles are left in the ears until the patient has achieved four consecutive weeks of abstinence or wants to drop out of the program. In another program, the needles are placed for thirty minutes at a time.

Another common site for acupuncture is on the surface of the nose, which is supposed to decongest the respiratory tract and generate a feeling of disgust for smoke.

A new, more modern form of acupuncture involves lasers. Laser beams are focused on the ear, nose, and a spot between the index finger and thumb. The frequency with which laser treatment is used depends on the clinician doing the procedure.

How It Works

The method by which acupuncture works is not well understood by modern science. The theory behind the technique is that all human physical or mental problems, including addictions such as smoking, are due to energy imbalances. Often the body needs help with realignment or redirection of this energy. The placement of needles in strategic positions facilitates this realignment.

There are very few carefully done studies of acupuncture for smoking cessation. One study reported an initial 88 percent success rate for patients treated with needles in their ears. In this study, however, there was no comparison group. The patients reported to a clinic every week and were encouraged to quit. There is no description of the patients who participated in the study. As a result, it is impossible to evaluate how successful this program really was.

However, a more recent study recruited patients through advertisements and then randomly assigned them to three groups—one receiving no special treatment, one using nicotine gum, and one receiving acupuncture treatment. After one year, the researchers found that both the gum and the acupuncture worked better than no special treatment. Interestingly, the nicotine gum and the acupuncture seemed to work equally well.

Some studies have taken smokers and placed needles in the correct acupuncture site in half the group and in an incorrect site in the others. These studies have not consistently shown any benefit of acupuncture, but the numbers of people studied were very small.

This lack of conclusive information about acupuncture leaves the value of this technique in the speculative category. No one knows for sure whether or not acupuncture helps. There is a need for more definitive studies.

Harms

Acupuncture may seem harmless enough, but the small needles and staples have occasionally caused problems. Needles used in acupuncture are generally not disposable, and the same needles may be used repeatedly for different people. There have been reports of infections caused by unsterilized acupuncture needles. These infections may be at the site of the needle, or bacteria introduced into the bloodstream may cause an infection at a distant site (such as the heart). Also, acupuncture needles have transmitted disease from client to client. Cases of hepatitis have been transmitted between clients, and it is at least theoretically possible that even AIDS could be transmitted. As a rule, professional acupuncturists, ones who carefully take care of their equipment, do not have these problems. But if you wish to try acupuncture, be sure you find a reputable practitioner who sterilizes needles between uses.

An understandable concern for those considering acupuncture is pain. Most practitioners claim that acupuncture is a relatively pain-free procedure. (We guess "relatively" is the key word!) Some people have reported some discomfort, either during or, in some cases, after the procedure. Considering that pain is a uniquely experienced phenomenon, it's up to you to decide if you'd like to further pursue this technique.

Recommendation

Acupuncture can be recommended only with reservation. Although it may attract many smokers looking for something new, conclusive evidence to support its use is lacking. Nevertheless, it is accepted by some experts as possibly helpful, especially with supportive counseling and proper smoking-cessation strategies.

Make sure you know about the training of the practitioner, his or her method of sterilizing needles, and the satisfaction of previous clients who have used the treatment (and the particular practitioner) to try to stop smoking.

HYPNOSIS

Clinical hypnosis, in general, involves the induction of a deep state of relaxation during which a subject is more receptive to the power of suggestion. Hypnosis is supposed to remove or restructure subconscious ideas and attitudes that prevent success and, hopefully, accentuate those that will enhance it.

When it comes to quit-smoking programs, however, hypnosis can mean almost anything. There is no standardization of technique. In addition, anyone can claim to be qualified. As a result, the experience and expertise of the hypnotist can vary widely. Skeptics believe hypnosis to be pure magic; many other people see it as having great scientific potential.

How Is Hypnosis Used?

How does hypnosis help smokers quit? Some hypnotists give a single session for one person. In this session, the hypnotist may teach you to hypnotize yourself and, thereby, maintain the effect. Other hypnotists require you to attend more than one session.

Typically, a smoker is instructed to use this self-hypnosis many times a day. This approach is intended to help the smoker develop a positive, receptive attitude toward quitting.

Some programs employ group hypnosis. It has not been demonstrated that the success of this approach differs from that of individual sessions. Nevertheless, the medical literature contains some studies reporting good success rates for some group hypnosis programs incorporating counseling, strategies, and support.

Follow-ups are usually recommended in hypnosis programs if a person wants to continue to remain smoke-free.

Finally, there are programs that are promoted as hypnosis but do not actually use it. These programs use the mystique of the word to attract the attention of smokers. This is why you need to be an informed consumer.

Self-Hypnosis

Many people are confused about the difference between hypnosis and self-hypnosis. There is actually very little difference. Hypnosis uses the talents of a hypnotist, but this person is actually teaching you to hypnotize yourself anyway. In self-hypnosis, you hypnotize yourself to achieve your goals, using skills you have learned from reading or from a professional.

Some people respond better when they are guided by a professional. In quit-smoking programs, knowing that a professional is experienced and has had good results can add immeasurably to the confidence you have in the program. But you'll still want to continue self-hypnosis procedures to maintain your results.

Hypnosis most frequently incorporates positive, motivating suggestions designed to increase the smoker's confidence and strength to quit. The following are some examples of the suggestions used.

- "I will feel better and healthier as a nonsmoker."

- "Smoking is a poison to my body."

- "I need my body to live."

- "I am in control."

- "I enjoy being a nonsmoker."

These, and many others, are suggestions that, when heard while you are in the deeply relaxed state of hypnosis, become part of your new belief system. With repetition, these suggestions overcome and replace the negative attitudes that have helped you maintain your smoking habit.

In addition to positive suggestions, hypnotic procedures often include relaxation and imagery to help you stop. Imagery involves creating pictures in your mind in a way that reinforces your desire to quit. Common images focus on seeing yourself as a nonsmoker; seeing how proud, confident, and healthy you are when you go to functions and are not smoking; and the healthy state of your body (and mind!). You can create any images that are significant for you.

There are many different approaches to hypnotic suggestion. Other than the positive suggestions mentioned before, some hypnotists may use aversive therapy, giving strong suggestions to the subject that he or she will experience an unpleasant sensation while tasting or inhaling cigarette smoke. Suggestions also focus on the idea that the smoker will no longer enjoy smoking. Research has indicated, however, that positive, constructive suggestions work better than negative, aversive ones.

Effectiveness

Hypnosis may be effective in helping you in a few different ways. It can be used to remove subconscious barriers to success. Also, the mystique surrounding the technique may increase your confidence in your ability to quit. If you believe in hypnosis, then its effect on you can be very helpful. Unfortunately, not every smoker can successfully be hypnotized (although a vast majority of all people, if they are willing, can). Of the smokers who can achieve a deep level of hypnosis, many seem able to quit. Among the others, the results vary.

In scientific circles, there is dispute over the value of hypnosis in quit-smoking programs. Hypnosis seems to work best when it involves several hours of ongoing treatment with a therapist who tailors the session to the smoker's individual needs. The success of these programs may be as much due to the attention given the smoker as it is to the particular technique itself. The variety of programs that employ hypnosis makes it difficult to precisely state its effectiveness. There is difficulty in distinguishing the sham operation from a well-designed program run by a sincere, talented practitioner. Some programs appear promising, but few good studies of the method have been published. If you are interested in hypnosis, then you need to find a reputable program.

Where do you find a reliable professional or program? Check with your physician, local medical and psychological organizations, hospitals, or health organizations. The credentials and experience of the practitioner should be as important to you as those you seek for any other health-related purpose.

There are a number of questions you should ask about any hypnosis program that you are considering. These include: How reputable is the practitioner? How long has he or she been practicing? Where was he or she trained? Satisfy yourself that the hypnotist you are considering is an expert in the technique and that he or she uses the technique professionally and wisely. A recommendation from a reliable source is critical in this difficult-to-evaluate area.

What hypnotic suggestions are used? Does the program punish you for thoughts of smoking or encourage you to overcome subconscious hurdles? You want to make sure that the approach being used, whether positive or aversive, is one with which you are comfortable.

How long does the hypnosis program run? Although a single session will be cheaper, more sessions seem to be more effective.

Is there any long-term follow-up? What does the follow-up cost? Find out all possible costs at the beginning. The more you know, the more comfortable you'll be. The last thing you want is to have additional expenses sprung on you. This may make you feel that unless you fork over the extra cash, you'll have to stop the program in midstream, leaving you unsuccessful.

What are the program's success rates? Phenomenal rates (70 percent or greater) should concern you as much as low rates. Remember, there are no guarantees for success. (Be wary of any program that offers one.) Also, find out when these success rates are calculated, since they are always higher rate after the program ends than they would be one month or one year after completion.

There are some programs that say you can continue at no extra charge until you successfully complete your attempt to stop smoking, and you may want to consider them more favorably. Ask if you can have the names of some former clients, although confidentiality may be an issue in some cases. Often, though, successful clients are very willing and eager to brag about their accomplishments.

Concerns About Hypnosis

Many people don't even consider hypnosis because they are afraid of it. But their fear usually stems from a few common myths. Let's briefly discuss these. Remember, as you read, that all of these myths are untrue.

Myth number one: Hypnosis is all theatrical entertainment.

The truth: Professionally done, clinical hypnosis is totally different from entertainment hypnosis.

Myth number two: You're out of control when you're hypnotized.

The truth: You're completely in control at all times. Your good judgment continues to be in effect. You will not do anything under hypnosis that you would not normally do.

Myth number three: You are asleep during hypnosis.

The truth: You are awake and alert, although your body is in a relaxed, restful state. You have to be awake in order to hear the suggestions that can make you a nonsmoker!

Myth number four: You will experience amnesia.

The truth: You'll remember everything that occurs during the procedure. If you forget anything, it might be the same type of minor details that you'd forget about a movie you just saw.

Side Effects

There are very few side effects with hypnosis. People unfamiliar with it are usually wary of the technique. Reading about the procedure (there are many good books available) can help. Experts state emphatically that neither the technique nor the practitioner can force someone to do something against his or her will and that the technique is generally safe. The most important adverse effect of a hypnosis program is what it can do to your pocketbook. Investigate all the costs before you sign up for any program.

A COMMENT ABOUT TAPES

There are dozens of tapes on the market that deal with hypnosis for smoking cessation or just giving up smoking itself. Beware. You never know (until you listen) if you'll find the voice relaxing.

A voice that sounds like nails on a blackboard would hardly be conducive to success! Also, using a tape requires a certain degree of self-discipline in order to incorporate the included techniques. Further, you don't know if these techniques are what you need anyway.

So yes, tapes may be helpful, but the number of possible disadvantages warrant careful investigation before choosing a tape. And, of course, use the tape as *part* of your total stop-smoking program.

Recommendation

Hypnosis may indeed make a contribution to helping smokers quit. The best practitioners have moderate success—especially when hypnosis is combined with other methods. This technique cannot (and should not) be dismissed as worthless. Further studies of its effectiveness are needed. Meanwhile, if you are interested and are having trouble with other methods, hypnosis may be worth a try. At best, it may be very helpful. At worst, it is most likely harmless.

ONE FINAL NOTE

There are other techniques that may also contribute to the deconditioning process. Relaxation and meditation, for example, can reduce stress and eliminate obstacles to quitting. Many successful programs include these techniques. You may choose to include them in your quit-smoking package as well.

CHAPTER 10

The Physically
Aversive Strategies

Making Smoking Physically Unpleasant

Most smokers find smoking a pleasurable activity. Each puff provides a reward for continued smoking. It supplies the body with the nicotine it craves. It provides pleasure in meeting your habitual needs and cravings (both physiological and psychological).

A basic premise of why we do what we do is that the consequences of our behavior either sustain or reduce the behavior, depending on whether the consequences are pleasant or unpleasant. Since a pleasant experience is what causes you to sustain smoking, one strategy to help you quit is to make smoking as unpleasant as possible. This approach pairs smoking with unpleasant thoughts, feelings, tastes, or sensations. Hopefully you'll develop an aversion to cigarette smoking. This should, as a result, make it easier for you to quit. Both this chapter and Chapter 11 review methods of "aversive conditioning"—the process of making smoking unpleasant.

MEDICATION

There is one medication that is used for the sole purpose of making smoking unpleasant. This product, silver acetate, has been marketed for decades as an over-the-counter medication to help smokers quit. Although it is not used commonly in the United States, it is popular in Europe.

Silver acetate is unlike products such as nicotine gum that are designed to ease physical withdrawal symptoms. This medication is intended to make your life uncomfortable when you smoke. The goal is to associate an unpleasant taste with cigarettes, breaking the connection between smoking and pleasure. (In addition to silver acetate, there are a number of mouthwashes, lozenges, and other smoking deterrents that are made from silver nitrate, copper sulfate, or potassium permanganate. Drug companies, though, have not rushed to make these products available to the consumer.)

History

Silver preparations were successfully used to deter adolescents from smoking over fifty years ago. However, the use of silver has never been popular in the United States.

Preparation

Silver acetate is available as a gum, mouthspray, or tablet, though it is most commonly administered as a chewing gum. Each piece of gum contains 6 milligrams of silver acetate as well as sugar, colorings, flavorings, and a gum base.

How It Works

This medication works by clinging to the surface of your mouth and producing a distinctly disagreeable metallic taste whenever you smoke.

Proper Use

Smokers are usually told to chew the gum for thirty minutes, six times a day, for three weeks. The gum is not recommended for use for more than three weeks and should be avoided completely by pregnant smokers (but so should cigarettes). The usual strategy is for smokers to continue smoking for the first week with the gum and then to quit smoking during the second week. The first week creates the association between smoking and an unpleasant taste. Continued use of the gum will hopefully deter you from going back to cigarettes.

Side Effects

Some people have concerns about exposure to silver. However, it is a metal that causes few health problems in humans. Cases of silver poisoning are extremely rare and the doses used in silver acetate gum are generally considered safe.

However, the drug has produced a few side effects. In a study of smokers in South Carolina, silver acetate was found responsible when about 1 in 6 smokers complained of side effects concerning their mouth (including bad taste connected with food, dry mouth, and a green tint to the tongue). About 1 in 8 using silver acetate gum complained of nausea, heartburn, or abdominal cramps. But of the over 150 smokers who used the silver acetate gum, only two stopped using it because of the side effects.

The most feared side effect of silver is argyrism. This strange-sounding condition is a permanent bluish-black discoloration of the skin, eyes, and mucous membranes that occurs with chronic exposure to silver. The discoloration occurs first in areas exposed to light. If the silver is not discontinued, it will soon spread throughout the body. There is no danger to your health with this condition, although the discoloration can be upsetting.

There have been at least two related reports of argyrism. In one report, the smoker took a very large dose of the gum over a period of six months. In the other, the smoker took the correct dose but continued it for two years. Because of the rare occurrence of this type of problem, almost everyone, including the FDA, considers silver acetate gum to be safe.

Effectiveness

How effective is silver acetate gum? That's an important question. Authorities in this country generally do not endorse silver acetate as an effective aid to smoking cessation. For instance, the FDA has stated that, although silver acetate gum is safe, there is not enough evidence to conclude that it is effective.

It is difficult, however, to completely dismiss the claims of advocates of silver acetate. At least four studies suggest that it may help smokers. In particular, the South Carolina study found that the initial success rate among smokers taking silver acetate gum was 11 percent—almost three times higher than in smokers chewing gum without silver acetate. In this study, the smokers received no special instructions or counseling. Four months after the end of the study, the success rate among those who had used the silver acetate was 7 percent. Though this was low, it was almost twice as high as that of the comparison group. The smoking status of the participants was confirmed with a special blood test. These results suggest that the silver acetate gum was successful.

However, a recent important study from Denmark could not confirm this effect. This investigation was completely different from the South Carolina study. All the participants attended group counseling sessions at which lectures, support, and advice about quitting were given. In addition, the study compared silver acetate gum, nicotine gum, and ordinary gum as aids to smoking cessation. Almost 500 people who had smoked at least half a pack of cigarettes a day for the previous five years were enrolled in the study. What was remarkable was that after one year, the success rate was over 23 percent. This is much higher than in most other studies. This success was attributed to the effect of the group sessions. Nevertheless, there was no difference in success found between the group that chewed nicotine gum and the group that chewed silver acetate gum. Even more surprising is that the results of these two groups were no different than those of the group that chewed ordinary gum.

The experience with silver acetate is a good example of why it's so hard to say definitively that a certain product is beneficial in helping you to quit. Various studies, conducted under different conditions, often reach opposite conclusions. Because of conflicting findings about silver acetate, there can be no consensus about the role of this medication in a smoking-cessation program.

Recommendation

Unlike some medications, such as sedatives and lobeline, there is some modest support for silver acetate. The good news is that its side effects are more bothersome than dangerous and it is unlikely to cause harm.

If you would like to try silver acetate, the best we can say is "good luck." It may be worth it after other methods have failed.

SMOKE-AVERSION TECHNIQUES

If you enjoy smoking, then maybe too much of a good thing will help you to quit. At least, that is the theory behind the following smoke-aversion techniques. These techniques involve oversmoking in the hope that this will turn you off of cigarettes. The idea is to repulse you with too much cigarette smoke. By forcing you to inhale much more smoke than you normally do, the chemicals and gases in the smoke impact on you in an increasingly uncomfortable way, in some cases to the point of vomiting. At first thought it may seem extreme to make yourself ill from cigarette smoke in an attempt to quit smoking. However, these techniques have many advocates and have been widely studied.

Let's discuss a few of these aversive techniques.

Rapid Smoking

Rapid smoking is a technique that requires you to inhale from a cigarette every six seconds until either the entire cigarette is finished or you feel nauseated. You are to continue this rapid smoking until you are unable to take another drag. If you are able to continue, you should do so for a particular period of time, such as eight to ten minutes. During the session, you are to focus on the unpleasantness of the experience.

Rapid smoking is a type of procedure that should be done only under proper medical supervision because of the possible side effects. Programs are most often organized into six to eight supervised sessions. This is a good idea because of the need for supervision.

As part of an organized program, rapid smoking may be a helpful technique for some people. Studies show that some smokers do develop an aversion to cigarettes after a few sessions. Programs that have combined rapid smoking with other behavioral techniques have had the best results. Some report that as many as half of the smokers who used this program are still successful after a year. *The 1988 Surgeon General's Report* states that "the weight of evidence suggests that rapid smoking by itself can have a substantial immediate effect on cessation." But most experts recommend that you not try this technique on your own.

Satiation Smoking

In this strategy, smokers are instructed to double or triple the number of cigarettes they smoke and to keep smoking the increased number until they're no longer interested, usually because they have become ill or bored.

An early report about satiation found that more than half the smokers in the program remained abstinent after four months. However, no other study has come close to these findings. The biggest problem with satiation is that smokers are usually expected to do the program themselves in unsupervised settings. Even the most motivated smokers may have trouble increasing their consumption of cigarettes to the point of illness. Consequently, the effectiveness of this program, and its ability to produce an aversion to cigarettes, is questionable. Nevertheless, some authorities still advocate satiation and feel that it is good preparation for quitting.

Blown Smoke

This is one of the first smoke-aversion techniques, reported initially in 1964. It merely involves blowing warm, stale smoke in the faces of smokers while they are having a cigarette. You can probably imagine why this technique is not one of the more highly regarded ones!

Other Programs

Many other forms of smoke aversion have been tried. One program, called forced chain smoking, had smokers smoke eight complete cigarettes in a row in six sessions each. In another program, participants drew a large puff of smoke into their mouth and held it for thirty seconds while focusing on the unpleasant sensations it caused.

Effectiveness

Many of these techniques were promising when they were first introduced, but only rapid smoking continues to have strong support.

Side Effects

The side effects of techniques that increase the amount of smoke you inhale are a potential problem. Rapid smoking can significantly raise your blood pressure and heart rate. Your exposure to carbon monoxide decreases and can further impair your body's ability to deliver oxygen. Rapid smoking can also cause abnormalities in your electrocardiogram. Nevertheless, despite these effects, the technique is safer (if you stop!) than a lifetime of continued smoking. Because of the effects on the heart and lungs, the technique is not recommended for individuals with known cardiac disease, diabetes, or disease of the lungs or blood vessels, unless administered under close medical supervision. None of the techniques should be used if you are pregnant or if you suffer from congestive heart failure. If you have any questions at all as to the adverse effects of these techniques on your health, be sure to speak to your physician.

Recommendation

If you want to try a smoke-aversion technique, find an organized program that uses rapid smoking. The best, most effective programs seem to schedule six to eight sessions and use other behavioral techniques as well.

PAIN TECHNIQUES

There are other forms of aversive conditioning that involve pain or discomfort. These approaches take the idea of making smoking unpleasant to an extreme. Let's discuss two of the techniques.

Shock Therapy

This may be hard to believe, but shock therapy has been used as an aid to smoking cessation. This shows just how desperate some smokers are to quit. In this program, an electric shock is paired with smoking as a punishment. The goal is to help the smoker develop an aversion to cigarettes. Research has shown that programs such as these do poorly in comparison with other stop-smoking programs.

Rubber Bands

A milder form of pain technique is the use of a rubber-band snap. Smokers in this program are instructed to wear a thick, loose rubber band on their wrists and to painfully snap the rubber band every time they have the urge to smoke. Rubber-band snapping should continue until the urge to smoke fades. It should not be done so intensely that it breaks the skin or leaves welts! Rather, it is designed to "jolt" you into distraction so you'll temporarily focus on something other than smoking.

Effectiveness

The effectiveness of pain techniques is far from proven. Punishment is seen as the primary motivator to quit smoking. It's as if you're saying, "I'll stop smoking so I can stop the punishment." Research has been far from convincing in its investigations of punishment as a technique. Punishment seems to be unpredictable and varies too widely. These tactics do not seem to be very attractive methods of quitting. There should be stronger proof that they work before you consider submitting yourself to this extreme type of approach.

CHAPTER 11

The Psychologically Aversive Strategies

Making Smoking Psychologically Unpleasant

There are some programs that have used the power of the mind to develop an aversion to cigarettes.

One popular approach is to have smokers save their cigarettes in a water-filled butt-jar. They are asked to stare at the jar and concentrate on the unsavory aspects of smoking. This exercise serves to disgust, if not nauseate, some smokers.

Another popular technique is called thought stopping. Whenever you get a thought about smoking, yell out the word "stop!" (Be careful, of course, that you don't do this in a crowded, public place!) If there are people around, *imagine* that you're screaming the word out. Or imagine a big red stop sign, or a great flashing sign that says "stop." You'll be trying to scare the thought of smoking away.

Some people find that this technique works even better if they do it together with another aversive procedure, such as the rubber-band method mentioned in the previous chapter or banging a heavy book down on a table.

In some programs, smokers are asked to focus on the unpleasant aspects of cigarettes as they smoke. They are supposed to think about the irritation of their mouth and lungs, the coughing, and the accumulation of smoke on their clothes, in their house, and in their lungs. In other programs, smokers are encouraged to use their imagination to develop an aversion to cigarettes. For instance, smokers might imagine being poisoned as they smoke and can envision escape from danger when thinking of not smoking.

Do you want to try something scary? Take a drag on your cigarette but don't inhale. Keep the smoke in your mouth. Now place a clean, white handkerchief over your mouth and blow the smoke through it. What do you see? The discoloration in the handkerchief is from the tar in the smoke. The amount on the handkerchief is approximately the same as the amount you deposit in your lungs every time you inhale. Imagine what your lungs look like (and how their function is affected) by inhaling just one complete cigarette. And what about two, or three, or a pack, or . . . Scary? Yes it is. Learn from this!

Why are aversive techniques like these used? The purpose is to increase your resolve to succeed in quitting cigarettes. Sure, you may admit that smoking is harmful to your health. But are you really aware of the degree of risk or damage? Or do you push these thoughts out of your mind? Some people feel that focusing on negative images of smoking and on its consequences can help turn them off to smoking.

WHY DO SMOKERS DENY?

Most smokers are aware that smoking is a health hazard. Nevertheless, there are gaps in their knowledge. Part of the problem is that they do not often want to acknowledge the harms of smoking. A 1987 survey revealed that 30 to 40 percent of smokers do not believe that smoking increases their risk of having lung cancer, other types of cancer, heart attacks, stroke, or lung disease, or that quitting would lower their risk.

When you smoke, you tend not to think about the bad effects. That's natural because it helps you to be able to keep smoking without feeling guilty or uncomfortable.

NEGATIVE VISUALIZATIONS

Using imagery to get a good, clear picture of the unpleasantness of smoking is a popular aversive technique used in many programs. However, studies do not clearly indicate how successful this technique is. Experts say that those who use it, though, can increase their chances of success. Let's follow a typical visualization procedure. Try to vividly picture what will be described to you. If you do not want to use this technique, then you may want to skip the next several paragraphs.

As soon as you inhale your first cigarette, the damage begins. The "wonderfully delicious" smoke starts attacking and corroding the mucous membranes of your eyes, nose, tongue, gums, mouth, throat, and esophagus. It moves on to attack your lungs, heart, circulatory system, and virtually every other part of your body now being "nourished" by impure smoke and chemical-filled oxygen. The chemicals in smoke remain with you (even after you exhale), affecting all of your important organs. Also, it is said that the radioactive contents for a pack-a-day smoker are equivalent to that of taking several chest X-rays each year.

You are inhaling addictive, toxic substances that can ultimately cause a number of different diseases and possibly even premature death. In addition, cigarette smoke contains many harmful substances that damage your lungs and deprive your body of oxygen. These toxic substances include a number of dangerous gases, such as carbon monoxide, ammonia, and hydrogen cyanide, among others. The smoke damages your lungs directly. The poisons, once absorbed into the bloodstream, injure your body's organs. Over fifty of the ingredients contained in cigarette smoke cause cancer.

You're also inhaling oodles of tar. Sounds delicious, doesn't it? Tar contains over thirty different cancer-causing agents (carcinogens). Even with low-tar cigarettes, you inhale more tar than your lungs are designed to handle. Besides, inhaled smoke decreases the effectiveness of your lungs to handle things (tar, dirt, microbes) you really don't want cruising around in your lungs, which serve in a protective capacity. Any time an "intruder" gets into your lungs, these protective agents move it toward your throat, from where you can cough it out. But if smoke damages your protectors, the bad guys remain in your lungs. Sorry, pal.

Every one of the 50 million Americans currently smoking is being harmed by the use of cigarettes. Imagine the damage you are inflicting on your body. You'll seem to age faster than non-smokers. This aging affects your appearance (more wrinkles) as well as your lung function. You'll develop more respiratory-tract infections. You may have a chronic cough and develop annoying hacking. Aside from bad breath and discolored teeth and fingers, you may lose your ability to taste. You may even recover from many illnesses at a slower rate than do nonsmokers. And, imagine the horror of knowing that you could get cancer, heart disease, or lung disease, in addition to many other problems, including peptic-ulcer disease, stroke, and osteoporosis.

Remember: focus on the fact that every cigarette harms you. Every cigarette burns in smoke that can cause danger to the functioning of your body. Can you imagine yourself going to your medicine chest and drinking poison? No? So why smoke it?

THE EFFECTS OF SMOKING ON NONSMOKERS

Now that you've distastefully pictured how smoking can damage your body, think about how exposure to environmental tobacco smoke can be dangerous for nonsmokers as well.

Smoking doesn't just harm you. As a smoker, your habit and addiction affects others. Imagine the fumes from a cigarette wafting their toxic gases toward those who are with you, those you care about. Your loved ones are breathing in your smoke. This can be as damaging as if they themselves were actually smoking! This is called passive smoking.

Can you imagine your loved ones developing cancer, chronic lung disease, or any of the other smoking-related medical problems? This can be a successful aversive technique for many smokers. You may not care about hurting yourself (or even believe that it's going to happen), but what about your loved ones? There is no doubt that smoke from cigarettes causes harm, no matter who inhales it.

You can't forget about your children, either. Children *do* suffer from environmental smoke. Children of smokers grow more slowly and experience more physical problems and symptoms than do children of nonsmokers.

Further, if you are pregnant, you might want to consider this. As a smoker, you are reducing your chances of a successful pregnancy. Smoking sabotages nature's attempt to provide a safe place for the development of the fetus. Pregnant women who smoke are more likely than nonsmokers to have a miscarriage, and complications during pregnancy and labor are more common.

The problem is that toxins from cigarette smoke enter your circulation. These substances, like nicotine, flow freely through the placenta and into the fetus, poisoning the developing fetus. Babies born to smokers may comprise 20 to 40 percent of all low birth-weight infants—those at highest risk for health problems.

SHOULD YOU USE AVERSIVE TECHNIQUES?

Using the physiological and psychological aversive techniques mentioned above may be harder than other techniques. It's certainly easier to pop something such as a pill or Nicorette gum into your mouth. But if you work with a technique that clearly reminds you of the damage smoking can do both to your body and to the bodies of your loved ones, you may have a much stronger desire to enhance your health by quitting.

There is currently no strong evidence that aversive techniques can help you quit smoking. But, it is certainly valuable to focus on the positive aspects of life without cigarettes. These types of techniques, involving pain and thought power, can all be considered types of punishment. The problem with this is that in general, aversion techniques, if they work at all, only seem to be effective for the short term. They leave a lot to be desired. However, in some cases, they can be useful, especially if they set the stage for a continuing effort on your part.

A NOTE ABOUT BEHAVIORAL TECHNIQUES

Aversive techniques are a type of behavior modification. "So," you might say, "what about some of the positive behavioral techniques that are designed to make things more pleasant as a nonsmoker?" Well, these procedures are very important. In fact, practically every successful quit-smoking program recommends that behavioral procedures be part of the package. Examples of successful self-management procedures include relaxation, desensitization, and behavioral rehearsal. We will discuss a number of effective behavioral strategies in upcoming chapters.

Part III
Quitting!

CHAPTER 12

Working Alone or With Others

Once you have decided which program or techniques seem best for you, the next important step is to determine exactly how you're going to use them to become an ex-smoker. There are three main ways to implement your program. You may choose to do it on your own, with individual counseling, or in a group. All three, or any combination, offer you different possibilities in your quit-smoking program.

SELF-QUITTING

Most smokers try to quit on their own. More people have stopped smoking by using a self-quitting, cold-turkey approach than by using any other method. Usually when people stop cold turkey, they set up their own method of quitting. Smokers who prefer this approach often choose to quit without the help of a formal program.

You can implement most of the strategies that we've discussed without a formal program. You might want to obtain brief instructions on how to quit and then follow them on your own.

If you're quitting on your own, then your most vital need is information. This book provides a lot of the basics, but don't feel that you have to stop here. There are plenty of other good sources that you may want to consider. The best place to start is with nonprofit organizations because they usually have an abundance of good material that is available free or at a minimal charge.

Where to Get Information

There are a number of national organizations that can be valuable resources. Here are just a few of the better-known organizations. Addresses and telephone numbers for each of them is found in the Appendix.

National Cancer Institute

The National Cancer Institute of the National Institutes of Health is a great place to start. With just a phone call, this government agency will send you many helpful pamphlets. There are people available there to talk to you about smoking-cessation programs. In addition, they have lists of programs located in many parts of the country.

American Cancer Society

The American Cancer Society (ACS) is a voluntary organization composed of 58 divisions and 3,100 local chapters. Through the Great American Smokeout in November, the annual Cancer Crusade in April, and many educational materials, such as the I Quit Kit, the ACS helps people learn about the health hazards of smoking and how to become successful ex-smokers. They also sponsor the Fresh Start program, described later in this chapter.

American Heart Association

The American Heart Association (AHA) is a voluntary organization with 130,000 members (physicians, scientists, and laypersons). AHA produces a variety of publications and audio-visual materials about the effects of smoking on the heart. It has also developed a guidebook for incorporating a weight-control component into smoking-cessation programs.

American Lung Association

As a voluntary organization of 7,500 members (physicians, nurses, and laypersons), the American Lung Association (ALA) conducts many public information programs about the health effects of smoking. The organization actively supports legislation and information campaigns for nonsmokers' rights. It provides help for smokers who want to quit, for example, through Freedom From Smoking, a self-help smoking-cessation program available in most cities. It also provides materials and guidelines to help people stop smoking and remain ex-smokers.

Office on Smoking and Health

The Office on Smoking and Health (OSH) is the Department of Health and Human Services' lead agency in smoking control. OSH has sponsored distribution of publications on smoking-related topics, such as free flyers on relapse after initial quitting, helping a friend or family member quit smoking, the health hazards of smoking, and the effects of parental smoking on teenagers.

Hotlines

Many communities offer hotlines to help smokers who are trying to quit. There are many advantages to hotlines, including being free of charge and accessible to anyone with a phone. These programs offer personal contact without the face-to-face interaction that may discourage some smokers from joining a more formal program. A recent study of ten counties in western New York State found that a hotline significantly increased quit rates.

Hotlines may be helpful. Check in your community and find out if there is one available. Even if you do not use it, it may be useful to have the number available—just in case.

Social Support

The presence of a partner or other social support can often make the difference between success and failure. Many people who quit on their own have actually relied on the encouragement of others. Don't be reluctant to recruit others into your effort. Sure, you're the one with the ultimate responsibility for quitting, but others can help get you through the tough times.

A recent study suggests that partners can contribute by being supportive and that their positive behaviors can help you quit. These behaviors include, for example, complimenting you on not smoking, congratulating you for your decision to quit, and participating in activities with you to help keep you away from smoking.

On the other hand, the study showed that negative behaviors by partners were not helpful. These behaviors include, for example, commenting on your lack of will power, mentioning being bothered by smoke, criticizing your smoking, or expressing doubt about your ability to quit. In fact, there is some evidence that these negative comments can even neutralize the benefits of the positive ones.

What should you do? Tell your partner and friends what will help you. Enlist their positive support.

Individual Counseling

The chances of success with virtually any program can be enhanced by counseling. Counseling can help you increase your knowledge about why you should stop and how. Counseling may also help you learn more about why you haven't yet been successful in giving up cigarettes.

Individual counseling is an alternative to self-quitting. There are a variety of health professionals trained in behavioral modification techniques applicable to smoking cessation. Many of these counselors also teach stress-reduction techniques.

All too often, physicians assume that their patients know everything they need to about the hazards of smoking and the techniques for quitting. This, unfortunately, is often not the case. Counseling by health professionals can help ensure that you have the necessary information.

The most important aspect of individual counseling is the counselor. Therefore, your efforts should be focused on finding someone who is recommended. Contact nonprofit institutions (for example, hospitals or the ACS) for referrals. Once you are referred to a professional, ask any essential questions to assure yourself that this is someone with whom you want to work. Make sure you ask about the counselor's credentials and training. Inquire about the techniques used in smoking cessation, how much experience he or she has, and what the success rates have been. You may also want to find out how the professional deals with obstacles to success. You might even ask if you can speak with people who have used this counselor.

GROUP PROGRAMS

Group programs are a way in which you can get support from others who are also attempting to quit smoking. Working with them through organizations or nonprofit clinics can be very beneficial. Often, getting involved with such organizations will enable you to have low fees, leaders who have been trained in relevant areas, and heavy emphasis on health education. This combination can be very valuable in helping you to stop. Often, organizations such as the AHA, ACS, and ALA have programs such as this.

There are many different methods employed by groups. They may be as diverse as the different types of people who participate. Your choice will probably be influenced by the content and style of the program as well as its cost.

In general, group programs increase your chances of success. The biggest problem with many formal smoking-cessation programs is that so few smokers take advantage of them. And you might not even be aware of some of the best, most effective programs.

Studies show that only about one in twenty smokers use an organized group program to stop smoking. While these programs may not always produce dramatic results, they do contribute to helping smokers quit.

Formal Organized Programs

Virtually every city has organizations, both nonprofit and for-profit, that offer quit-smoking programs. Many of these programs are advertised in the Yellow Pages, in newspapers, and at community meeting places. Some programs are unstructured, while others follow a rigid agenda. Many incorporate methods that are discussed in this book, including nicotine gum, hypnosis, and behavioral methods. Some last less than a week; others go on for months or years. Many are offered at a nominal fee; others carry a hefty price. Most of the programs consist of a series of classes or group meetings. A few require that you reside at a facility to immerse yourself in the quit-smoking process.

A variety of programs are described in this section. They give you an idea of what's available, though they are not the only ones. Virtually every community has some variation of these basic programs.

Freedom From Smoking

The ALA sponsors an excellent program called Freedom From Smoking. It is a highly structured program that focuses on behavioral change. Its underlying premise is that smoking is a learned habit that must be unlearned. It is also a cold-turkey program. You are expected to quit completely, soon after the program begins. You should be ready to make the commitment before you start this type of plan.

Freedom From Smoking usually includes seven sessions that stretch over seven weeks. Each session takes about two hours. The first few are scheduled at weekly intervals. The third is called Quit Night and all participants are expected to have quit smoking by that time. Within forty-eight hours of Quit Night, another session is held to help participants through the roughest days. Then one session is held in each of the following two weeks, followed by a two-week interval and the last session. Each session typically includes some opening words by the group leader, and then the participants break up into discussion groups.

Sessions focus on how to quit. There is not a lot of time spent talking about the dangers of smoking. Various helpful techniques are discussed. The program is designed so that smokers can help each other quit. Group interaction is considered a very important part of the program.

The Freedom From Smoking program is not meant for half-hearted participants. The group leader tries to discourage smokers who are not truly motivated to quit. It is thought that participants who are not ready can demoralize others in the group.

The program currently costs less than $100. The fee is considered a sign of your commitment to quit.

How successful is the program? A survey revealed that one in five participants was free from cigarettes at one year. Many of those who failed had been unable to quit even during the seven weeks of the program. Of the smokers who quit during the program, the ALA says that almost four in ten were able to stay away from cigarettes in the following year.

Freedom From Smoking is an excellent program, offered throughout the United States, for a motivated smoker who responds well to group situations. It was designed and organized by professionals and seeks to help you help yourself. It applies most of the proven methods mentioned in this book.

Five-Day Plan or Breathe-Free Plan

This is one of the most popular, widely used nonprofit programs in the world. The Five-Day Plan was developed by the Seventh-Day Adventist Church and is available through hospitals, churches, and companies around the world. This plan not only has helped more than 14 million smokers in over 150 countries but it has also served as an example for the development of similar programs.

The program originally had five structured classes that met on consecutive days, plus several follow-up meetings. After a few revisions, the program is now called the Breathe-Free Plan to Stop Smoking and involves eight sessions given over three weeks. However, the original principles have been retained. One of the reasons the program was extended is that smokers often need the most help over weekends, and it was felt that a course that lasted over three weeks could help get the quitters over the first few Saturdays and Sundays. The charge for the program is determined at each location, but it is usually very low.

The sessions typically begin with a film showing surgery on a cancerous lung. Participants are expected to stop smoking on the third session. The first session is an introduction to the program, and the second is a preparation for quitting. After the third session, the classes emphasize the harms of smoking and provide information on diet and various relaxation techniques so that you may begin the maintenance phase of a smoke-free lifestyle. Speakers in the program may include psychologists, clergymen, and physicians. They all emphasize the philosophy of the Breathe-Free

Plan to Stop Smoking, which is to empower you to reach three major objectives: physical preparation, mental conditioning, and social support.

Regarding physical preparation, the program assists you to begin and maintain an exercise program, to break free of all drugs or habits that impair judgment, and to learn to improve your diet. The mental conditioning is designed to help you think like a nonsmoker and to replace the physical urges to smoke with plans that can help the mind overcome the physical addiction. Finally, the social support is designed to help you avoid friends who smoke and drink, smoking family members, and office parties where tobacco may be present, and to learn to counter tobacco ads by telling yourself the truth about tobacco. The program also emphasizes the value of networking with individuals and groups that support a smoke-free lifestyle. Information about this program can be obtained by calling 301-368-6718.

Fresh Start

The ACS runs Fresh Start, another excellent and popular group program. This program, provided through the over 3,000 chapters of the ACS, is commonly offered in the work place. It costs about forty dollars, although it may be less if your employer contributes. However, the ACS suggests that employers not pay for the entire program since the cost may provide an incentive to the smokers to take the quit attempt more seriously.

The program, organized as five one-hour sessions given over about four weeks, is designed to provide you with information and strategies that can help you succeed. Participants meet in groups of eight to fifteen people. The leader tries to get the participants actively involved.

In the program, the participants discuss topics such as addiction, stress management, withdrawal symptoms, quitting methods, weight-control strategies, and how to avoid returning to cigarettes. In the first session, you explore your smoking habit. You fill out four questionnaires designed to determine if you really want to change your smoking habits, what you think are the effects of smoking, why you smoke, and whether your environment will help or hinder your attempt. You are also asked to designate a quit date, which is expected to be within the first week. The other sessions are organized to provide you with practical skills that will help you to succeed.

Other Group Programs

There are also many commercial, for-profit programs advertised to help you quit smoking. Because it is so difficult to develop a successful program, however, many have gone out of business.

Smoke-Enders is perhaps the best known of all the commercial programs designed to help smokers. It was started in 1969 by housewife Jacqueline Rogers, who, after giving up smoking, decided to make a business of helping others to do the same. The program claims that its goal is not only to help you quit smoking but also to help you enjoy not smoking and be comfortable as a nonsmoker. The philosophy of the program is that the more responsibility you take for changing your life, the more successful you will be. They claim that they have had 800,000 graduates of their program and that they are currently seeing approximately 10,000 to 15,000 smokers a year.

Smoke-Enders is organized as a series of six weekly meetings of about two hours each. The program consists of a wide variety of presentations on topics such as the nature of addiction and the effects of nicotine. There are also significant group discussions. The program is based on nicotine fading and participants are allowed to smoke for the first four sessions. This is an important distinction from any other program in that you are not expected to go cold turkey on the first day of class. Buddy groups are often set up during the Smoke-Enders sessions. These groups may continue to meet after the class has ended. Smoke-Enders is available to individuals in most states, and many companies also offer the program. Its base price is $325. The company says that you may repeat the course, if necessary, for half price, if you are unsuccessful in your initial attempt. One of the nice aspects of Smoke-Enders is that it aims to help you concentrate on increasing your motivation to quit by visualizing a sense of personal gain rather than self-denial and resentment. The literature specifically states that the group does not use techniques based on fear of health hazards or death. It does not use scare tactics, guilt producing images, shock treatments, or hypnosis, and no medication is given or prescribed.

Smoke-Enders' literature claims that of 4,000 recent graduates, 84 percent indicated that they are not smoking at one year after completing the program. This figure seems too good to be true, but it is likely that Smoke-Enders has helped a significant number of people to quit. For those who do not have access to the Smoke-Enders program, there is an audio-cassette program, which takes you through eight weeks rather than six weeks. It currently costs $125. To reach someone at Smoke-Enders, you can call toll-free 800-828-HELP.

The concern with commercial programs is that the costs are high. Some people question whether or not the profit motive interferes with helping people to stop smoking. Although there are a few studies of the commercial programs, it is clear that programs like Smoke-Enders are based on sound principles. Despite high fees, many people have found them helpful. Besides, having to pay higher fees may increase your motivation since you probably do not want to waste your money.

Spas

If you have the financial resources, a spa is one place you can go to quit smoking. Spa programs usually combine counseling or behavior modification with a beautiful setting designed to ease your transition into quitting.

Newsweek recently gave some publicity to the spa approach. It carried a report about a smoking treatment center that operates out of Palm Springs Spa Hotel in Florida. For a mere $350 a night, you can check into the program and be pampered by herbal baths, massages, gourmet meals, and eucalyptus-inhalation therapy. In addition, the program includes group counseling and constant attention from "chemical dependency counselors."

Some spas transplant a traditional program into a very pleasant setting. An example of this type of program is at Saint Helena Hospital, just north of San Francisco. This spa program, run by the Seventh-Day Adventist Church, offers the Breathe-Free Plan to Stop Smoking, which we discussed earlier in this chapter.

Because of the expense of these programs, very few people use this approach to quit smoking. Many more, however, might be willing to spend the money if they knew these programs were effective. The important question is whether this approach works.

Unfortunately, there is very little information about the effectiveness of spas. And even if they do help you quit while you enjoy the idyllic environment, there is no evidence to suggest that this method will help you sustain your determination. Nevertheless, some people may consider these spas to be an excellent opportunity to combine a vacation with a smoking-cessation attempt. Therefore, if you have the money, it might be worth a try!

Effectiveness of Group Programs

There are many different types of clinics or organizations that sponsor quitting programs. These programs vary widely in procedure and may have benefits for motivated individuals. Unfortunately, they often have very high drop-out rates and their low success rates may not be encouraging. Because there has been very little scientific study done on these programs and their results, one has to take the success rates they publish with a "grain of salt." On the other hand, group programs may provide "just what the doctor ordered" for individuals who don't have the motivation or discipline to stop on their own. Of course, it takes discipline to continue attending a group program!

The effectiveness of these groups and programs varies tremendously. The skills of the group leader may determine why the program is successful in one locale and unsuccessful in another. Furthermore, the different programs emphasize a variety of approaches. There is currently no consensus that one approach is superior to another. Many programs have published their success rates. Unfortunately, they do not compare their rates to a similar group of smokers who did not participate in their program. A review of nineteen major programs revealed that the median quit rate one year after the program started was 25 percent.

Two researchers examined the Breathe-Free Plan. They found that when the program ended, a very high percentage of the participants had quit. Unfortunately, when they checked on these participants six months later, only 11 percent were still not smoking. A program similar to this plan, except that it also included personal telephone contacts, had a 34 percent success rate one year after the end of the program. Among all the reviews of this program, the success rate ranged between 20 and 30 percent.

Another recent study compared the two popular programs from the ALA and the ACS. This study enrolled over 1,000 smokers from three different communities. Overall, the Freedom From Smoking (ALA) program fared better than the Fresh Start (ACS) program. For both programs, the success rates after one year ranged from 10 to 20 percent. Although these results sound disappointing, they may be two to four times higher than what people achieve on their own. These results are very accurate because they were obtained by a team of researchers that has no interest in inflating the numbers. The numbers are more realistic than many of the amazing "unconfirmed" success rates claimed by some organizations. The results show just how difficult it is to quit. The good news is that at least one in five smokers who participated in these programs was able to become free of cigarettes.

When you are investigating a particular group or clinic to determine if it is worthwhile for you, the following questions may be useful.

Who runs the program?

A reputable organization, such as a local hospital or the ACS, will usually run a solid program.

Is the program primarily educational, is it unstructured, or does it contain a rigid plan for quitting?

You need to find a program that fits your needs. Since no program has been shown to be superior to the others, you should choose an approach based on your preference. The goal is to increase your confidence in your ability to quit. Decide whether you'd prefer an educational program or one that follows a very set quitting plan. Your decision may be partly based on the time you have available, the strategies used, and the relative costs of the programs.

Does the program provide for additional sessions once it is finished?

A good program will provide follow-up sessions to help you confront the possibility of relapse. Ask if the program does this and how.

What are the program's success rates?

A good program should be monitoring its success rates. Furthermore, you want to know how many people quit by the end of the program and how many remain ex-smokers one year later.

What does the program cost?

There are many good, inexpensive programs. You should not have to pay much for quality. On the other hand, some smokers are more highly motivated if they spend a significant sum for a quit-smoking program. Decide for yourself what will help you most. Also, you want to know if the program has a policy for refunds (not always necessary or even motivating) and what the costs might be for follow-ups or retaking the program. (For example, some good programs will allow you to take the whole program again for free, if you don't succeed the first time.)

Are the techniques used practical and effective?

You don't want to get involved with a program that uses weird, unproven techniques. Most effective programs use at least some of the techniques discussed in this book.

Try to find smokers and former smokers who have used the particular program you're interested in and were taught by the current instructor. Their comments will give you more of a feel for the program.

Most experts endorse the use of group programs to help you quit. No particular program has emerged as the single best one. If you are the kind of person who enjoys a group setting and would benefit from the mutual support of individuals in these groups, then you should definitely consider this option.

Although it is difficult to state precisely the usefulness of group programs in helping you to quit smoking, a well-organized group with an enthusiastic leader will almost certainly increase your chances of success. If you are the type of person who benefits from group support, and many do, then these programs may help you. They can be a source of information, support, and long-term encouragement.

THE PHYSICIAN'S ROLE

Regardless of whether you're going to stop on your own or with others, your physician may have an important role in helping you to quit. Let's talk about how physicians can be helpful in stop-smoking programs.

The best physicians for smokers are supportive and knowledge-able about smoking cessation. They do not try to scare their patients into quitting. That doesn't mean they avoid talking about the health risks. Rather, they discuss these risks in a way that can be motivating. These discussions also emphasize the benefits of quitting. They listen to their patients and help them develop personalized strategies. In addition, these physicians do not abandon their patients, regardless of whether or not they succeed in their effort.

Work with a physician who is qualified to help you. Inquire about the physician's interest and expertise in helping smokers to quit. Be assertive. Why? Because you need someone who under-stands the importance and difficulty of the task. Furthermore, you need a physician who knows the most recent information about quit-smoking methods. There are many who are very helpful resources for smokers who want to quit. Physicians who take a few minutes to discuss quitting with their smoking patients can dramatically increase quit rates. Even brief advice from a suppor-tive, qualified physician may help. The effect of this advice will be even greater if you are a smoker who has already developed symptoms or a health condition related to smoking.

Physicians with knowledge about quit-smoking methods are in a good position to help find suitable methods for you. Further-more, some medications that may help you quit require a physi-cian's prescription. Finally, a physician can be available to meet with you to help prevent relapse. Quitting is a long-term en-deavor. Your physician can be a great source of support.

CHAPTER 13

Your Comprehensive Program

You've been spending time reading about, and selecting, which program or techniques you want to use and determining if you want to quit by yourself, with a professional, or with a group. You should now have some pretty good ideas as to how you want to proceed. So the final step in your preparation is to develop your own personalized program. You're ready. And remember: you can succeed!

The key to your success is to have a plan. Because there is no one right way to quit smoking, you must put together your own best package. As you know by now, there is an abundance of different legitimate methods from which to choose. Mix and match methods if you want. It doesn't matter if you reject most of them, but make sure you select the methods that are best for you.

Before you take another step, make sure your stop-smoking plan answers the following questions: What will you do when you want to smoke? How will you cope with withdrawal symptoms? Will you try brute will power or behavior-modification techniques? Do you want to try it alone or with the support of others?

There are plenty of options. Review all the strategies and techniques available and consider your own needs. Be open to the idea of using a number of smoking-cessation programs or strategies. Don't feel that you should use only one. The more techniques you use, the more you increase the likelihood that you can succeed. Decide what's best for you as you develop your plan. Taking control of the situation is an important step toward success.

Don't be too concerned about the cost of your program. The more it costs you in terms of both involvement and financial considerations, the more motivation you will have to use the program and actually stop. Besides, you will be more than compensated for the money you spend—by the money you'll save when you're no longer buying cigarettes!

DEVELOP YOUR PROGRAM

Regardless of what specific program or techniques you use, there are a number of other strategies that successful smoking-cessation plans often include. Let's go over the essentials you'll want in your program.

Pick a Date

Once you know that you're ready, the next important step is to select a quit date. "There's never a perfect time to quit smoking," you're probably saying. Maybe so, but you'll want to find the best time for you. Pick the day carefully. Consider everything that's going on in your life. Try to select a time when you will not be stressed by other events. (Or, if you're *always* stressed, try to select a time of less stress than usual!) Don't pick a time when you have exams, a work project due, a family wedding, or anything else that is unusually stressful. Timing is everything.

Your quit date doesn't have to be today or tomorrow (although it can be, if you're fully prepared!). Pick a day within the next few weeks. If you're having a hard time deciding the exact date when you're going to quit, start by narrowing the range of possibilities to a longer time period first. For example, select two months. Resolve to yourself that, during that time, you'll pick the date that will be your quit date. Set the date at least one week away from when you finally make your decision. This will give you some time to prepare—and to psyche yourself as well.

Since timing is so important to quitting, you may want to consider a certain special day to quit. For example, if it is close to a loved one's birthday (including your own) or a holiday like Thanksgiving or New Year's, then those days might be appropriate. If you are ready to quit in the fall, you may want to target the Great American Smokeout, which takes place each year on the Thursday before Thanksgiving. This is a national event, sponsored by the ACS. It's designed to provide the greatest national support for smokers thinking about quitting. On this day, every smoker is encouraged to give up cigarettes.

As the Great American Smokeout approaches, information about quitting is distributed at schools, worksites, and healthcare facilities. Newspapers and magazines are filled with articles about smoking cessation. Every smoker is encouraged to participate and to abstain from smoking for as long as he or she can. This is a good opportunity to join others throughout the United States.

The idea for a national quit-smoking day began in the 1970s. In 1972, the ALA in Oklahoma sponsored a no-smoking day, and the ALA in Minnesota soon followed. In 1977, the ACS formally initiated the Great American Smokeout.

The program has been very successful. According to a Gallup poll, 90 percent or more of the United States' population is aware of this program. More importantly, in recent years, over 10 percent of all smokers did not smoke on this day and approximately 30 percent more reduced their total number of cigarettes.

Many people use the Great American Smokeout as a springboard to long-term success. By making the Thursday before Thanksgiving the focus of your efforts, you can feel like you belong with thousands of smokers across the country who will also attempt to free themselves from cigarettes on this day. (And, on Thanksgiving, you'll have a great reason to be thankful—you will be an ex-smoker for a week!)

The relative calm on the date you select should extend beyond your quit date. You want the calm to extend through (as much as possible) the period of the following day as well. For example, you might want to consider quitting during vacation time. Some people do best when they don't have regular pressures on their minds. Others, however, may prefer to stay busy, figuring that will help to distract them.

Once you pick the date, circle it on a calendar, which you should put in a prominent place. As your quit day approaches, get rid of cigarettes, ash trays, and lighters, especially from the places where you spend a lot of time. On your quit day, wake up as a non-smoker. Focus all of your attention on *not* smoking that day. Tell anyone in whom you've chosen to confide about your plans to quit on this particular day.

Have your entire day planned. Keep busy. Make sure you

include some enjoyable activities. Do something special to celebrate this momentous occasion. Remind yourself of your transition from smoker to ex-smoker and what it means to you.

Remember: once you've set the date, *do it!* Don't procrastinate!

Monitor Your Current Cigarette Use

Knowing details about your current smoking behavior is another key to success. Monitor your smoking every day for a week. When do you smoke? How much do you smoke? What are your trouble spots? When do you crave a cigarette? What triggers your urges? How do you feel when you smoke? This will let you know your smoking patterns at the point at which you're starting your efforts to quit. It will also indicate the potential triggers for smoking and obstacles to stopping. Knowing this will help you to pay attention to those trouble spots that have the greatest chance of sabotaging your efforts.

Detail Your Reasons for Quitting

Do you know why you are quitting? Are you quitting for health reasons? Because smoking is simply not as socially acceptable as it once was and you want to avoid the social stigma of it? Because you want to save money? Or because your mother-in-law (brother, sister, parents, employers, etc.) told you to quit? These reasons are only the tip of the iceberg.

Remember, the motivating reasons for quitting must be your own. Smokers who succeed know why they quit. It's important that you are quitting for your own unique reasons, rather than because somebody else is telling you that you should. For example, you may know that quitting will reduce your chances of illness. But most people who smoke know that. So why haven't they all stopped? Because that simply may not be a sufficient reason! (By the way, this never ceases to amaze never-smokers, who can't believe people would continue to smoke despite the health risks.)

Take some time and sit down with a pencil and paper to write down every single reason you can think of for why you want to quit smoking. Reflect on the reasons that motivate you most. Be as specific as possible. Put this list where you will see it often so your reasons can encourage you. Add to the list as additional ideas pop into your head.

Some people choose to write each item on an index card, adding to their stack of cards as they think of an idea. Include ideas such as: "Smoking is a sexual/romantic turnoff." "Smoking can destroy my lungs." "Smoking makes my breath taste awful." "Smoking affects the other important people in my life."

Detail Your Expected Benefits

Smokers who succeed also have a clear idea of how they will benefit from quitting. Write down the benefits you expect to get, the same way you've already listed the reasons you want to quit. The more you'll benefit, the better you'll cope with the challenge. These benefits will be your reward.

Once you get past any withdrawal from cigarettes, you will feel better overall. Even if you do not currently suffer from any health problems, there are some immediate benefits for you. You'll be less winded with exertion, and you'll feel better about yourself!

List all the benefits you can think of. Do it right now. Hold on to your list and add each new idea to it. Some examples? If you are watching your pocketbook, then the money saved from not buying cigarettes may be important. If you have grandchildren, then a desire to see them grow up may motivate you. If you are a parent, you may not want your children to follow you into the habit and addiction of cigarette smoking. If you are an adolescent, you may want to avoid being ensnared in a life-long addiction to cigarettes.

If you used the index-card idea in the previous strategy, you might want to write the benefits on cards, too. In fact, write each benefit on the reverse side of the card, listing your reason for stopping. For example, on the back of the card that says, "Smoking makes my breath taste awful," you could write, "As a nonsmoker, my breath will taste clean and fresh."

Have you thought of quitting as something being taken away from you? That's negative thinking. Consider this way as an alternative. Think of giving up smoking as a remarkably powerful medicine that you are being offered. What can this medicine do?

Here is a sample list of benefits from some smokers who have successfully quit.

- I'll have more energy at work and on weekends.

- I won't be sick as often.

- My breathing will improve.

- I'll live a longer life to enjoy with my family.

- My home, clothing, and car will smell cleaner.

- I'll feel proud of myself.

- I'll be setting a better example for my children.

- I'll smell better (to myself and to others), and my breath will be better.

- My fingers will stop yellowing.

- I won't cough as much.

- Stopping will clear the stains on my teeth.

- I won't worry about getting cancer, heart disease, or other chronic illnesses.

- I won't have to hide my behavior from my family.

- I'll be rid of an unpleasant, unhealthy behavior.

- My athletic performance will improve.

- I'll live a longer, healthier life.

Look at Yourself in the Mirror and Tell Yourself You Can Succeed

Smokers who succeed in quitting have (or develop) confidence in their ability to do so. Look in the mirror and say aloud that you can quit. Say it often enough that you'll believe it more and more. The more you repeat these positive affirmations, the more you'll absorb them.

Keep giving yourself positive messages to keep your motivation high. Tell yourself such things as: "I am a nonsmoker." "I've succeeded in stopping; now I'm going to stay this way." "I am helping myself to achieve the health and peace of mind I want." Keep repeating these thoughts to yourself. It can be even more effective if you repeat them out loud.

Find Sources of Support—Family, Friends, Colleagues, Etc.

The more public you go with your efforts to stop smoking, the more positive reinforcement you can get from the people around you. The battle to become a former smoker is made easier with the support of friends and family. Enlist their help. Do not underestimate the importance of social support in your effort to quit smoking. Many studies have found that smokers who have the support of their family, partners, and friends were more likely to quit and remain abstinent. Research has shown that the more people you tell, the greater the likelihood of your success.

Some people feel that they don't want to tell anyone until they have quit. They want to surprise them. Unfortunately, the surprise is more often on the smoker, who goes back to smoking with those around him or her none the wiser! So let people know your intentions. Develop, and put in place, a support system before your efforts begin. Tell your friends when you're going to quit. Seek their support. In addition, after you have told everybody, do you really want them to see that you're having a problem? That concern may help to keep you on the right track.

Be honest with them. Warn them that you may be a bit more irritable than usual during your quit-smoking endeavor. If they're aware of this, it increases the likelihood that they'll be supportive. Otherwise, they might want to put you out to pasture! Tell them not to nag. Support and encouragement is one thing, nagging is another.

By the way, don't be discouraged if any of the people you tell don't believe you or doubt that you can succeed. Look at this as a challenge. You'll show them!

Quitting With a "Buddy"

The buddy system is another type of support. It can be very

helpful to quit at the same time as someone else. For example, at any sign of weakness, you know you have someone to give you that little extra strength that just may guarantee your success!

Using a Professional

Some people like working with a professional, such as a qualified psychologist or social worker. This person may help you to deal with any obstacles that may arise, as well as any stress or depression that may interfere with your progress.

Increase Your Physical Activity

Increase the amount of healthy activity in your daily routine. Strenuous exercise is not necessary to help you quit. Even a twenty-minute walk every day is beneficial. Use exercise as a way to relax, focus on health, and distract you from cigarettes. (Check with your physician if you have any concerns about including vigorous exercise in your daily routine.)

Eat Well (Properly and in Moderation)

We've discussed the fact that one of the problems some people have with quitting (and even anticipating quitting) is the tendency to gain weight. You do want to combat this, don't you? Steer your diet away from high-fat, high-calorie foods. Drink plenty of water. Lots of cool, refreshing water can strengthen your body and nourish it, and can greatly help you to reduce cravings.

Avoid Potential Triggers for Smoking

Minimize the number of cues or triggers that may remind you that you miss smoking.

Structure your physical environment to make it easier for you. Make your home and work place as smoke-free as possible. Make sure there are no cigarettes around at all. Any available cigarette may cause you to inadvertently light up and smoke before you even realize what you're doing!

Get rid of matches, other than a few that you might want to keep for lighting candles. Do you have any ashtrays or lighters that have sentimental value? If so, stash them. Get rid of any others or find new uses for them, such as holding candy or plants, or serving as coasters.

Change Behavioral Routines

For the period of time right after you stop smoking, change the routines that may interfere with your success. For example, if you are used to smoking while you talk on the phone, try to have briefer phone conversations. You'll only have to do this for a short period of time in order to break these habits. Another example? If you're used to smoking with a cup of coffee at mealtime, don't linger after you finish eating. Develop alternative plans. Avoid situations that are conducive to smoking, as well as people who make it difficult to be a nonsmoker.

Control Your Stress

Stress can be a powerful saboteur to your stop-smoking program. After all, it's one of the most common reasons people smoke. You'll want to do everything you can to reduce it and keep it from thwarting your efforts to quit. Knowing yourself, knowing when you're under stress, and knowing how to be in control of your stress are essential to any successful quit-smoking program.

To begin a stress-reduction program, start by identifying your stressors. (What is it that causes tension in your life?) Then determine if these stressors can be changed or if it's more reasonable to work on changing the way you deal with them. Either approach can help you to reduce stress.

Include peaceful, relaxing activities to give you a break. This also gives you the confidence that you, not stress, are in control. Examples of peaceful activities you can enjoy are quiet time, which you can actually schedule into your day; short breaks, or even naps; exercising, whether it's calisthenic or purpose-type (such as gardening, sports, or riding a bicycle); calling people with whom you enjoy talking; eating breakfast, lunch, or dinner with different people whose company you enjoy; and getting a massage.

Relaxation techniques can be very effective stress-controllers. Here's a quick introduction to one relaxation procedure called, appropriately, the *quick release*. Read the instructions first and then try it. Close your eyes, take a deep breath, and hold the breath as you tighten every muscle in your body of which you are aware (your fists, arms, legs, stomach, neck, buttocks, etc.). Hold your breath, keeping your muscles tense, for about six seconds. Then let the breath out in a "whoosh" and allow the tension to drain out of your muscles. Let your body go limp. Keep your eyes closed, and breath rhythmically and comfortably for about twenty seconds. Repeat this tension-relaxation cycle three times. By the end of the third repetition, you'll probably feel a lot more relaxed.

Decide which stress-controlling activities are most suitable to your needs, and use them. The list is limited only by your imagination.

Rehearse and Visualize Having Your Last Cigarette

One of the most important factors in being successful as a non-smoker is for you to be able to clearly picture your life without cigarettes and recognize this change as being a very positive one.

See yourself as a nonsmoker. Determine when you're going to stop and see yourself as a nonsmoker from that point on. Prepare for smoking that last cigarette. Decide in advance when it's going to be. Close your eyes and visualize the experience. Visualize, as well, the period of time immediately after you stop. See yourself facing new situations without cigarettes. The more frequently and vividly you visualize this culminating step, the more likely it is that it will occur just as you visualize it!

Envision yourself in different situations in which you have smoked in the past. See yourself in these situations as an ex-smoker. In order to succeed, you must prepare for the eventual obstacles, temptations, and urges that you will be experiencing. Rehearse the strategies that you'll use in difficult situations so that when they occur, you'll already know how you're going to deal with them.

Make a Contract

Making a "contract" with yourself or others is often an effective way to help yourself quit. For example, you might want to make up a formal contract that contains your quit date with a vow to stop smoking. Decide exactly what you intend to accomplish and write it down. Put it in the form of a contract, either by yourself or with a supportive person. State explicitly when you will quit and how you will do it. Sign the document in the presence of a witness, and stick to it! This may help you strengthen your resolve to avoid cigarettes.

A few smoking-cessation programs hand out such contracts on the first day. You might want to hang your contract in a prominent place to remind yourself of your commitment to quit. Remember, every bit of commitment is a step towards success.

A variation of this idea would be to make a bet with someone. Set it up, though, so you are the only one who can lose. And then, don't lose!

Another idea might be to make a contract with someone that includes a monetary incentive. People often respond to rewards for certain behaviors. Some formal programs collect money from smokers during the first few sessions and repay the money depending on their ability to remain abstinent. There are other variations on this theme. One of the more powerful ones has had smokers donating money to an organization or political candidate that they do *not* favor for each cigarette they smoke. What a punishment! Or, they may commit to doing chores that they would like to avoid.

Substitute More Appropriate Activities

You may have a free mouth, free hands, or some free time at your disposal when you stop. Make sure you've planned on appropriate substitutes to get you through this initial difficult time. Such substitutes as chewing gum, fruit juices, and sugarless sucking candies can help the free mouth. Toothpicks, paper clips, or rubber bands can help the free hands. And activities such as exercising, bathing, reading, walking, or even watching television can help fill your free time.

Don't replace one bad habit with another, though. Fattening foods are not a good idea, and watch out for alcohol (more about that in the next chapter).

Round Out the Package

Decide what other tips or strategies you will use to supplement your basic program. There are a lot of additional things you can do, every one of which can increase the likelihood of your success. They include the following:

- Those things that you're going to do as replacement activities during the first, most difficult days should be readily available. If you are going to read, chew gum, do needlepoint, assemble jigsaw puzzles, or do anything else, have the materials out and available so that you can easily use them as a distraction.

- Go to the dentist and have your teeth cleaned. Get rid of yellow teeth, and have those sparklers increase your determination to keep them that way!

- Establish a savings account. Put all the money you would have been spending on cigarettes into this account and save it to buy yourself something special. After all, you're the one who is committed to quitting. Why not benefit in ways besides "simply" better health and longer life?

- Consider yourself, now and forever, a nonsmoker. (And, of course, don't do anything to change your status.) Put signs up in your house and office that say things such as, "Thank you for not smoking."

- Tell yourself, "I'm not going to smoke today!" For some people, the thought of never smoking again can be very frightening. Convincing yourself that it is a day-to-day change can make it a lot easier to take.

- Reward yourself. Buy yourself little treats, or do special things to remind yourself of the important goal you're achieving.

- "Fumigate" your car and home. Clean them thoroughly to get rid of all the smoke smells (and ashes).

There are many additional techniques that can be used to increase the likelihood of your success. Consider them. Only you know what techniques to try next, because only you know what's best for you. Choose the methods that appeal to you.

Be fully prepared with your maintenance strategies even before you stop smoking.

AND NOW . . . QUIT!

You've prepared a personalized program that makes use of the best information currently available about how to quit smoking. You've picked a date, reviewed your reasons for quitting and your expected benefits, and monitored your current cigarette use, with special attention to the situations that make you want to smoke. You've discussed your plans with a physician and have enlisted family, friends, and coworkers as sources of support. You're engaging in some form of regular physical activity, are eating well, and have signed a contract to quit smoking. In addition, you have considered the merits of other techniques, including nicotine gum and groups or clinics, and have decided whether or not to add them to your program. You have not embarked on this project casually. Your preparation and hard work should inspire confidence in your ability to succeed. You're on your way.

Now that you have all of your components in place to stop smoking, you're ready to do so. But once you stop, you will want to remain an ex-smoker. The next chapter will help you with the critical subject of relapse prevention.

CHAPTER 14
Preventing Relapse

Let's assume, at this point, that you've stopped smoking. Congratulations! But we want to keep it that way, right? So you need to maintain what you've already accomplished—being an ex-smoker. What's the key to succeeding with any quit-smoking program? Properly using maintenance strategies after you actually stop smoking. Without successful maintenance, no smoking-cessation program can be effective.

At this point, it matters less what specific techniques you actually used to stop. What matters more are the specific techniques you're going to use to remain an ex-smoker.

One of the hardest things about stopping is that this addictive habit is associated with practically everything that goes on in your life! Yes, that makes it hard to stop. But now that you have, it is essential for you to be prepared to break the hold this habit can have on you.

Success in quitting cigarettes comes in stages. When you first quit, be proud of yourself! You deserve it. Give yourself credit for this first victory. But remember: the battle does not end at one week, one month, or even one year.

As good as you may feel about having stopped smoking, you must accept one very important thing. Just as an addict always remains one step away from returning to drug use, anticipate that you will always be susceptible to the temptation of cigarettes. Although you do not smoke, as an ex-smoker, you will continually be enticed by cigarettes. Cravings and urges may still hit you at any time. You must be prepared. Your vigilance in avoiding cigarettes cannot end after the first few weeks if you intend to achieve long-term success. Once you quit, your new focus must be to avoid relapse.

WHAT IS RELAPSE?

Relapse is the term applied when ex-smokers return to smoking. This is the important area that is often neglected in discussions of quitting cigarettes. Sure, many smokers can quit for short periods of time. However, it is common to hear of people who have stopped and ultimately go back to smoking. They have relapsed.

The Two Components of Relapse

There are two main things that have to happen for there to be a relapse. First, there has to be a trigger, whether it's a problem, an emotion, stress, a social crisis, or anything else. And second, your ability to cope or deal with this trigger has to be inadequate or unsatisfactory. To prevent relapse, either of these two conditions has to be eliminated or avoided. You know very well that you can't simply avoid all triggers. That would be nice, but it just doesn't happen. So the main focus of your efforts has to be to identify potential triggers and improve your coping ability for each and every one.

Relapse Is Very Common

Have you ever experienced relapse? If so, you're far from being alone! Many people quit several times before they stop permanently. In fact, Mark Twain is said to have coined the phrase, "Quitting smoking is not so difficult. I have done it myself over a thousand times." This is not meant to be an excuse for you to relapse. It is very important that you do not become depressed if you do resume smoking. Rather, you want to be more motivated to try to stop again.

Be positive. Quitting for any length of time is a big accomplishment. Even one day is better than nothing. It shows you have the potential to stop longer. What relapse means is that you need to find a more effective strategy, one that is better for you. Hopefully, you'll learn from the experience.

It may seem like we're preparing you for failure. We're not. But we recognize that some people who are not adequately prepared for success do relapse. So don't be discouraged or feel like relapse is inevitable. The key word is preparation. The better you prime yourself for quitting, the better position you will be in to prevent relapse. The hard work you did to quit must be applied to keeping you away from cigarettes for the rest of your lifetime. Learning more about it will greatly improve your chances of success.

Who Relapses?

There is no way to accurately predict who will remain an ex-smoker and who will resume. No specific characteristic, whether it be age, sex, number of years smoking, cigarettes smoked per day, number of previous quit attempts, or smoking satisfaction, can help us correctly predict who will succeed and who won't. Surprising, isn't it? Relapse usually has nothing to do with whether or not you have stopped on your own, with program assistance, or with the help of other people. Everyone who quits smoking is at risk for relapse.

Why Does Relapse Occur?

What are the factors that may make somebody start smoking again? Once you quit, many things may conspire to bring you back to cigarettes. The temptations to smoke persist for a long time. Even months, years, or decades after quitting, you may feel urges. These urges may be triggered by a sight, sound, or emotion. Sometimes they occur spontaneously. It is your ability to cope with these urges, and your level of commitment to remain free of cigarettes, that will determine your long-term success.

Relapse is particularly common during periods of emotional stress. Almost three out of every four smokers cite stress as the cause of their relapse. It may be that ex-smokers are vulnerable to the power of the cigarette when they feel depressed, anxious, or angry about other aspects of their life. In these periods, you may act impulsively, think less clearly, and undo all your good work. This also occurs commonly when you drink alcohol. These are times to be especially careful about resuming the use of cigarettes.

Maybe you're under social pressure to resume smoking, or you're having difficulty in a social situation such as a relationship, or maybe you're having a hard time emotionally. You may be most likely to have a relapse if you're experiencing excessive negative emotions such as anger, anxiety, or frustration.

If your self-esteem is lower than you'd like it to be, this may prevent you from having enough confidence to maintain your nonsmoking status. If you gain weight, you may feel that giving up smoking was not worth it. You may choose to go back to smoking in order to take off the weight you have put on or to keep yourself from gaining more.

Relapse also occurs because ex-smokers occasionally convince themselves that they can smoke "just one." Some investigators of smoking behavior call having a single cigarette a slip. The problem is that a slip may indicate the beginning of a relapse. One cigarette often leads to another. Not too much later, you may have resumed smoking regularly.

That first cigarette is often *not* followed by binge-smoking. The second cigarette, however, usually follows within a short time, whether it is a few minutes, hours, or weeks. Then there is a gradual increase as your rationalizations kick in and your discouragement about not stopping grows.

When Does Relapse Occur?

Relapse can occur any time, any day. Some people believe that most relapses occur within the first thirty days after quitting. This is not true. Some smokers go almost two months, if not longer, before returning to cigarettes.

You might ask, "When am I out of the woods? When will I feel confident that smoking is completely in the past?" The answer? Never! Unfortunately, there is no time after quitting when you are truly and permanently safe from the possibility of resuming. Some people go back to smoking even after decades of abstinence. The message? Stay in control, practice the coping strategies we'll discuss in this chapter, continue to plan for potential trouble spots, keep reminding yourself of the benefits of being an ex-smoker, and breathe a (clear) sigh of confidence.

Where Does Relapse Occur

You can fall off the ex-smoker wagon virtually anywhere, whether it be at work, at home, in restaurants, or at social events. If you have relapsed more than once before, then you probably know that relapse circumstances often change from one quit attempt to another. It's very difficult to predict accurately when you might have trouble. Nevertheless, there are three danger spots that deserve special recognition (and special caution) for all smokers: anywhere you drink alcohol, anywhere other people smoke, and anywhere you smoked previously. It is especially risky when you are around other smokers. In 60 percent of relapses, the first cigarette is not purchased but is borrowed (mooched, bummed!) from another smoker!

The Common Relapse Settings

Research has shown that relapse is most likely to occur in the following situations:

- When you're experiencing extreme stress, especially at work.
- When you're having trouble with an interpersonal relationship.
- When you're having an emotional problem, including depression, anger, or anxiety.
- When you're relaxing, such as after a meal, or in a social situation (especially if you're drinking alcohol).
- When you're around other smokers.

Prepare yourself to deal with each of these situations. Your new healthy status depends on it!

THE ROLE OF CRAVINGS

In order to prevent relapse, you have to be able to deal with the addiction that you have just given up. As you know, this addiction and the cravings that go with it are often both physical and psychological. Anticipate that you may never totally eliminate those occasional urges to smoke. The goal is for you to gain sufficient control of these urges so that they don't present a problem for you.

One of the problems about cravings is that any time you have a craving of any type, you may immediately assume that it is related to a cigarette. Any intense emotion that you experience may remind you that you have stopped smoking. Therefore, you realize that you no longer have one of your former coping strategies. The more you think about this, the more difficult it may be for you to remain an ex-smoker. Plan for these situations. Rehearse the strategies you'll use to deal with them when they occur (and expect them to, so that you're well prepared!).

THE ROLE OF CONFIDENCE

How well do you handle the situations in which you previously smoked? What is your response to the question, "Do I think I can stop smoking?" Smokers who answer positively, expressing a belief in themselves, not surprisingly have higher long-term success rates than those who answer negatively. Your beliefs, expectations, and confidence about your abilities in these situations are critical to your ability to succeed as a long-term ex-smoker.

HOW TO PREVENT RELAPSE

Yes, relapse can be avoided. You can successfully quit cigarettes. It doesn't matter what your level of addiction was.

Do you want to know a common factor enabling many people who stop to remain ex-smokers? They usually have learned sufficient coping skills to help them deal with any of the difficult situations that might previously have either triggered smoking or resulted in a return to smoking. So, in order to be successful in quitting, you need to learn (or build up) these necessary skills. You must learn how to deal with the urges, cravings, and pressures that might otherwise lead you to smoke. The only way you will have lasting success is if you are able to learn these skills. The more you prepare, the more you will learn. The more you practice in your efforts to remain a nonsmoker, the more likely it is that you'll remain this way.

THREE EXPECTATIONS

In order to maximize your chances of successful quitting and prevent relapse, you need to bring three expectations to your program: expect a challenge, expect temptation, and expect success. These expectations will guide you to a life free from cigarettes. They are essential not only in helping you to quit but also in maintaining your status as an ex-smoker.

Expect a Challenge

Although an occasional smoker can quit without much difficulty, most find the task to be a challenge. Anticipate that it won't be easy. You may face any or all of the following: social pressures, nicotine withdrawal, stress, concerns about weight gain, decreased job performance, problems in relationships with others, and nagging self-doubts. These are common experiences for most smokers as they become ex-smokers. Expect to experience these challenges and rise to the task. What's the best way to help yourself deal with these possible problems? Preparation! This is where your hard work pays off.

Occasionally, you may feel yourself slipping. You may become frightened, feeling that all your hard work is about to go down the drain. Maintenance can include having a good social-support network, engaging in an exercise program, and developing coping strategies. You'll have your own unique needs for how maintenance strategies can be helpful.

Expect Temptation

Your ability to cope with temptation may be the most important factor in maintaining your success. How you handle situations that entice you to smoke will distinguish you from those who have failed. But remember that there is a big difference between coping strategies and will power. Will power is sheer resistance to temptation. It represents power against power. The power to resist smoking usually falters after a prolonged temptation. Researchers have reported what seems obvious: will power to resist smoking is less effective than are coping strategies. Coping strategies, on the other hand, are more effective ways of successfully dealing with temptation.

Cigarettes may tempt you every day. Advertisements will continue to catch your eye. You may be walking down the street, flipping through a magazine, or sitting in a stadium when a familiar ad beckons to you. Cigarettes are legal, cheap, and easily available. You know where you can get them if you really want to smoke.

You will continue to see smokers (friends or family members may smoke), and they will tempt you (even without meaning to). As you inhale the second-hand smoke from these smokers, your body will remember the power of cigarettes.

You will continue to visit places where you smoked, as well as to experience familiar situations. These external stimuli may pressure you to resume.

There will also be internal temptations. Your body will feel strong physical and emotional urges to smoke. You may want to smoke to relieve this discomfort. Expect these temptations and be ready to resist. Rehearse how you will respond. This is another way in which you can prepare.

Expect Success

Smokers who believe in their abilities have a much greater rate of success. At this point, you have every right to expect it. You've quit and you have a strong interest in remaining an ex-smoker. You've pulled together the important components to maintain your new healthy status.

STRATEGIES FOR RELAPSE PREVENTION

There are many things you can do to prevent yourself from relapsing. As with smoking-cessation programs, some of them will suit your needs more than others. Review these proven strategies and use the ones you like. Many of these relapse-prevention strategies are the same as, or similar to, the strategies you read about in the previous chapter. But this chapter contains information on how you can use these strategies to make sure you remain an ex-smoker!

Expect the Worst

Prepare, prepare, prepare for the inevitable cravings, urges, and temptations. They will happen. Expect withdrawal symptoms. It may happen, even if you don't think you're physiologically addicted. The successful ex-smoker is the one who prepares for these things and is ready with strategies to "confront and conquer." And the unsuccessful smoker? That's the unfortunate person who says, "Well, I've quit. Now I don't have to think about it anymore." Wrong! You have to think about it. We're not telling you to be obsessed with cigarettes, but you need to think of what could cause you problems and prepare for it.

You may want to use behavior-rehearsal techniques. You can actually rehearse (in your mind or for real) what you will do in sticky situations. Behavior-rehearsal techniques can work very effectively if you do them with a supportive person. The more you practice, the more confident you'll feel in these skills.

Think about the situations that were problems in the past. Remind yourself of your previous typical smoking patterns. Remember your trouble spots. Don't let temptations catch you off-guard. Be consciously aware of those potentially difficult or threatening situations. What are the high-risk situations for you? What are the times during which you are more likely to be tempted to smoke?

Pull out the lists you made of reasons you decided to quit and why it is important for you to be an ex-smoker. Rewrite the list, possibly even adding to it, to reinforce the reasons in your mind.

Think of the strategies that are most helpful in each situation. Plan strategies that you will use for each and every one of them. The more you anticipate, the more you can control. For example, you might think about the reasons you quit or the benefits you expect. Maybe the image of smelly cigarette breath or fingers yellowed from nicotine will help prevent relapse. How about thinking of a friend or prominent person who has succumbed to a disease caused by cigarettes? Think about your children or other loved ones. Let thoughts about them strengthen you.

Use Your Lists

In addition to the list of reasons to quit, refer to your list of expected benefits. Read it, and remember what you expect to achieve. Emphasize the benefits that mean the most to you. Add those you expect in the future. Aim to achieve these benefits one day at a time.

Keep reminding yourself of your desire to be free of the power of cigarettes. Be prepared to use these strategies at times of temptation.

Talk to Yourself

Many thoughts, feelings, and concerns may float through your mind. Emotions such as anxiety, worry, frustration, and even depression may make it hard for you to avoid the temptation of cigarettes. So talk to yourself. Be your own best friend. Give yourself the vocal support you need to surmount these obstacles.

Say positive things to yourself. Reassure yourself that you can (and will) succeed. Remind yourself that you're focusing on one day at a time. Tell yourself what you'll do to deal with any obstacle that blocks your path.

Talk about problems. If you face a temptation, ask yourself, "What's going on here?" Then follow with, "What can I do to beat this?" Suggest strategies to yourself and select the one that makes the most sense.

Avoid rationalizations. Don't allow any excuse for smoking to sabotage your efforts. There can be *no* legitimate excuse for smoking—*none!* Squash any of these common rationalizations, such as, "One little cigarette can't hurt me." "I deserve a cigarette." "I'll stop tomorrow." "No one will know if I have one." Or even, "I can't take it any more. What's the point?" The point is you're an ex-smoker now. Keep it that way!

A very powerful way of talking to yourself involves projecting. In other words, ask yourself how you'll feel in the near future if you do (versus don't) smoke. For example, say to yourself, "If I have this cigarette now, will it really matter to me an hour from now?" Compare this to, "If I don't have the cigarette, an hour from now I'll know I'm still an ex-smoker!"

Use Imagery

You can conjure up images in your mind that can enhance your success and decrease the chances of relapse. For example, imagine all the hideous pictures or films you've seen of people suffering from smoke-related diseases. Contrast your previously gray, diseased, smoke-filled lungs with your new (as an ex-smoker), pink, healthy, smoke-free lungs. The more vivid the picture, the more effective this technique can be.

You can also picture how happy your friends and family will be when they see you as a nonsmoker. See the looks of surprise and admiration on their faces when you have that cup of coffee after dinner *without* a cigarette. See the look of satisfaction on your doctor's face when you tell him or her that you've successfully kicked the habit.

Use imagery also as part of rehearsal techniques to deal with potential trouble spots. For example, if you know you always liked to smoke while driving your car, picture clearly how nice it will be to drive in a clean, fresh, smoke-free car. You can even anticipate getting the urge to smoke and see yourself saying, "No, I'm a nonsmoker," with a big smile on your face!

Avoid the Triggers

You know the touchy situations that are most likely to cause you trouble. Avoid them (or at least as many as you can), especially early in your program. So what if you miss that smoky card party a few times? So what if you don't go out to eat with friends for a few weeks? If you know that these or any other situations have been clearly associated with smoking in the past, change your plans until your confidence is greater and your habit is history!

Learn how to deal effectively with those thoughts or ruminations that might inadvertently lead to smoking behavior. And use the stress-controlling suggestions you read about in the last chapter.

Escape Temptation

There may be times when you can't avoid a tempting trigger. But that doesn't mean you have to remain immobile and subject yourself to the torture of temptation. Move, run, escape! Take yourself out of the arena, clear your lungs, and feel the energy, confidence, and motivation flow back into you.

For example, do you usually smoke after meals? If so, try to get up immediately after you finish eating, brush your teeth, or go for a walk. If you always smoke while sitting in a certain chair and watching your favorite television show, then sit somewhere else or record the show and view it at a different time. If you're really desperate, go someplace where you know you're not allowed to smoke. These are just samples of the many effective changes you can make. Your log, discussed earlier, can help you to decide which triggers need to be "plugged."

Any craving is short-lived and will pass if you remove yourself from the situation. Is this copping out? Absolutely not! You are doing what you have to in order to achieve your goal.

Distract Yourself

When temptation is highest, and avoidance and escape are impossible, distract yourself. Distracting activities are examples of effective coping behaviors. These are activities that draw your attention away from the immediate temptation. You may cope with the situation by changing the subject or doing something completely different. A brisk walk (or any form of physical exertion), an invigorating escape, will help distract you from the cues that are tempting you. Changing locations can be very helpful. So can humming or talking to yourself.

You can use imagery to distract yourself. Imagine peaceful scenes. For example, you may be able to focus on a beautiful beach scene when you feel threatened by the urge to smoke. This will help you to maintain your abstinence. Imagine your next (smoke-free) vacation. Think of something beautiful and peaceful. Or think about something engrossing—a sporting event, a book you read, a movie you saw, or someone with whom you'd like to talk. This all keeps your mind off you know what!

Relaxation techniques can also be very helpful, both as distraction strategies and for stress management. Use the quick-release exercise mentioned in the previous chapter. Use this technique whenever you feel the urge for a cigarette. It will probably help you feel much more relaxed and much more in control. (You can use it for other nonsmoking-related stressful situations as well!)

Substitute

Replacing a bad habit with something that can temporarily ease the transition is a good coping strategy. Of course, many smokers fear that eating and gaining weight will be the substitute. As we discussed earlier in this book, you don't have to gain weight if you eat properly. Eat crunchy, low-calorie foods like popcorn, celery, carrots, or sunflower seeds, and drink plenty of low-calorie fluids. Chew sugarfree gum or use sugarfree sucking candies. You can also substitute minty toothpicks and play with items such as rubber bands or paper clips.

Enlist Social Support

Think about the important people in your life. Determine who will be an ally and really help you during moments of weakness. Make sure you also determine those people who, for whatever reason, will actually try to sabotage your efforts. Obviously, you'll want to minimize your contact with them.

Call on your support network. Don't be shy. Many of your family, friends, and coworkers will rally to help you. Don't feel like you have to do this alone. You can derive social support from family, friends, colleagues, or professionals, depending on who has the most meaning to you. Discuss your concerns and don't be afraid to ask for support.

How can friends or family help? Have them call you, regularly and frequently, to see how you're doing. Have them offer frequent words of support and encouragement. They may also want to do special things with you, both to distract you and to reward you for what you're accomplishing.

Be as public as you can be in telling people what you have accomplished. Get into the habit of telling people every day, "Today is another day that I'm a nonsmoker." You'll find that they'll expect you to say this, and if you don't, they may question you! Fear of a negative reaction may be just enough to help you remain a nonsmoker. In fact, let people know that they should *not* comfort you if you do go back to smoking. In this way, you'll anticipate their negative reaction if you relapse.

It's also important to continue to be socially active. The more socially isolated you are, the greater is the likelihood that you will return to smoking.

Maintain a Smoke-Free Environment

If you are surrounded by smokers, then you may find it especially difficult to quit. Similarly, if you continue to be around places and situations that you associate with smoking, you may also be headed for trouble. Try to make some changes, especially in the first few weeks after quitting. This can reduce the pressure on you to smoke. Obviously, you cannot eliminate all temptations. But, as we said, the more environmental triggers you can eliminate, the better.

This suggestion is not always easy to implement. For instance, you may have a big problem if your partner continues to smoke. It would be great if you could convince him or her to join you. Not only would you be able to eliminate a source of temptation in your home, but also you could be mutually supportive during the process. Otherwise, it may be very difficult for a smoking partner to help you quit.

It will probably also be necessary for you to learn to be a little more assertive. You'll need to be able to ask people around you not to smoke, or at least to delay smoking until you're not there.

There are other assertive things on which you'll want to work. You'll need to be able to refuse cigarettes when people offer them to you. You'll need to ask people to respect your wishes for a smoke-free environment at times when the temptation (not to mention the smoke) can be overwhelming.

Remember, being assertive doesn't mean you're being aggressive. It's simply your right to stick up for things that are appropriate for you, without hurting someone else. Think about it—are you really hurting someone else by asking them not to smoke?

Maintain a Positive Attitude

Believe in yourself. Believe in your ability to overcome these challenges. You have worked hard to prepare for your struggle to escape from cigarettes. You can succeed.

Do everything possible to maintain a good, positive attitude.

You *can* successfully quit! If you start doubting yourself or losing your motivation, it will weaken your chances for success.

Plan on taking life one day at a time. It can be very upsetting to say to yourself that you will never smoke for the rest of your life. It can be much more comfortable to deal with not smoking today. You'll focus on your ex-smoking goal for tomorrow when tomorrow comes.

Use Contracts for Confidence

When you feel tempted, remember your contract. You made a commitment to quit smoking. Reflect on the work you have done and the progress you have made.

Remember that writing a contract can be a useful technique, not only for stopping initially but also in maintaining your ex-smoker status. It's amazing how writing down a goal or promise, and detailing how it will be accomplished, can increase your likelihood of success.

How do people use contracting? Some people specify a certain reward that will be obtained if they keep from smoking for a predetermined period of time. Other individuals may specify a certain amount of money that is going to be paid to somebody else (e.g., some people may pay money to an organization they do not support) if they do not maintain their ex-smoker status. Yes, this is an aversive technique. But the goal is to do everything possible to help you to remain an ex-smoker.

Get Medical Feedback

Stay in touch with your medical professionals. Get information from them about your improved state of health since you quit smoking, specifically, information about your improved breathing capabilities or your increased ability to exercise. Physical examinations can be very motivating when they show that your health is improving.

Reward Yourself

Implementing a self-reward program can also be a good relapse preventer. Give yourself frequent and meaningful rewards for remaining a nonsmoker. This will help you to deal with those times when it may seem more desirable to return to smoking. Any rewards that are going to be used, however, must be significant to you. If they aren't, they will have no value whatsoever in helping you to achieve your goals.

Participate in Work-Place Incentive Programs

It can be very helpful to involve yourself in a program in the work place or with other individuals at work if no formal program applies. You may be able to receive incentives such as cash bonuses, prizes, or increased vacation time, or use other types of reward strategies that can help you to remain a nonsmoker. (Of course, if you're not working, there's nothing wrong with a "home-place" incentive program!)

Avoid Slips

Every ex-smoker is tempted to smoke from time to time. The downfall of many quit attempts begins when someone decides that he or she can smoke just one. As we explained, almost all smokers who have a lapse go on to full relapse. The lapse creates an opening for a return to full-time smoking.

If you feel that you are weakening and are convincing yourself that, although you want to remain an ex-smoker, you would like to smoke just one cigarette, merely to remember the taste or the feeling, *then freeze*. Stop and analyze the situation. You should smoke that cigarette only if you decide that you cannot continue as an ex-smoker and want to return to smoking. Make a conscious decision. Do not be at the mercy of an impulse. If you feel that these impulses are leading to a slip, get some help from a friend, a coworker, or a family member. Do everything possible to avoid the slip. Realize that the temptation will pass and consider how you will feel in a few hours if you allow yourself to smoke.

Once you are past the temptation, analyze what happened. Determine what was going on at the time to contribute to the potential slip. Develop a strategy to avoid finding yourself in a similar position in the future.

If you do slip and still want to remain an ex-smoker, do not despair. While it is true that 80 to 90 percent of people who have a slip go back to full-time smoking, there are exceptions. Just because you slip does not mean that you *have to* become a smoker. To succeed, however, you must reevaluate your commitment and plan how you will avoid the next temptation. This is an important time to use your support network.

Delay the (Unfortunately) Inevitable

There may be times when, despite all of your efforts, you just *know* you're going to have a cigarette. The craving may be too intense or your current situation may be too tempting. Don't just give in to it. Delay your lighting up as long as you can. Even though you smoked, knowing you delayed the act can at least reassure you that you have *some* control! This can help you get back on track.

There may be some times when your delay tactics work better than you anticipated. Cravings don't last forever, you know. A delay might get you past the cigarette you wanted, enabling you to continue as a successful ex-smoker.

Strengthen Your Body

You can increase the chances of maintaining success and preventing relapse by improving your nutrition and increasing exercise.

In order to minimize any physiological effects of withdrawing from nicotine, make sure that you eat a well-balanced diet. Improving your diet and including regular exercise in your routine will help you to deal with any physical or emotional roadblocks that may make it difficult for you to remain a nonsmoker.

Beware of Alcohol

Many relapses begin when judgment is impaired by alcohol. If you surround yourself with smokers and drink alcohol, then relapse is almost guaranteed. Don't be at the mercy of alcohol. It can weaken your resolve and can send you back to smoking even without your consciously deciding to do so. This warning does not mean that you must avoid alcohol completely but only that you need to recognize the risk it poses for your now healthier, cigarette-free life.

Conclusion

So now you're on your way. Use this book as your guide to success. You can do it. Before we close, let's throw a little more good news at you. Want to know the very best health news about giving up cigarettes? Quitting really does make a difference! Even if you have smoked for years (and years and years . . .), quitting can improve your health almost from the day you stop!

If you suffer from lung or heart disease, then you will benefit almost immediately by ceasing to inhale the poisons found in cigarette smoke. By avoiding your daily dose of carbon monoxide, your body will function better.

Quitting cigarettes is like a "wonderful medicine" that can prevent so many of your ills, begins working almost immediately, and benefits you more the longer you take it. Sounds too good to be true? It's not. When you stop smoking, you'll see for yourself!

But you're not the only one who will benefit from this. Everyone around you will derive direct benefits. This magic formula can improve youthfulness and prevent disease in you and those around you. No other single drug, vitamin, food, or activity can do so much to improve your health and help those around you.

WHAT DOES THE SURGEON GENERAL HAVE TO SAY?

There is now no doubt that giving up smoking will improve your health and help you to live longer. The 1990 *Surgeon General's Report* on "The Health Benefits of Smoking Cessation," in over 600 pages of studies, results, and documented findings demonstrating the health benefits of quitting, concludes that "smoking cessation has major and immediate health benefits for men and women of all ages." The report further states that "former smokers live longer than continuing smokers . . . [and that] smoking cessation at all ages reduces the risk of premature death."

Read for yourself the major conclusions of the report:

- Smoking cessation has major and immediate health benefits for men and women of all ages. These benefits apply to people with and without smoking-related diseases.

- Former smokers live longer than continuing smokers.

- Smoking cessation decreases the risk of lung cancer, other cancers, heart attack, stroke, and chronic lung disease.

- Women who stop smoking before pregnancy or during the first three to four months reduce their risk of having sickly babies, as compared to women who continue to smoke.

Aren't these benefits worth quitting for?

WHAT DOES THIS MEAN?

You're probably now asking, "Can I be sure that quitting smoking will improve my health?" The answer is an emphatic, "Yes!" There is no doubt among medical authorities that quitting will not only improve your health but will also decrease your chance of developing many deadly and disabling conditions. Even long-term and older smokers have the power to improve their health by quitting. Furthermore, the longer a person stays smoke-free, the more his or her health risks decrease, eventually approaching those of a nonsmoker. These studies form the basis of the aggressive quit-smoking campaigns that currently exist throughout the country.

Here's another great reason for quitting. More and more people are becoming concerned about the air around them. This applies both to people who smoke and people who do not.

The topic of environmental tobacco smoke (ETS) is becoming one of increasing concern for the public. Not only do you want to stop smoking so that you can do your part, but you also don't want those around you to be affected by ETS. More and more people are talking about the "smoke-free work place" and other smoke-free environments. This is your way to do your part to make these ideas become a reality.

WHEN DO THE HEALTH BENEFITS OF QUITTING BEGIN?

The health benefits of quitting smoking begin soon after you put out your last cigarette. Most quitters report feeling better almost immediately. This is not just a psychological feeling. Your body does respond immediately. To show you exactly what happens in your body after putting out that last cigarette, here are some significant statistics from the American Cancer Society.

Within twenty minutes of your last cigarette:

- the blood pressure drops to normal;
- the pulse drops to its normal rate;
- the body temperature of your hands and feet increases to normal.

Within eight hours:

- the carbon monoxide level in your blood drops to normal;
- the oxygen level in your blood increases to normal.

Within twenty-four hours:

- the chance of heart attack decreases.

Within forty-eight hours:

- nerve endings start regrowing;
- your abilities to smell and taste things are enhanced.

Within seventy-two hours:

- the bronchial tubes relax, making breathing easier.

Within two weeks to three months:

- the circulation improves and walking becomes easier;
- lung function increases by up to 30 percent.

THE VERY LAST WORD (WE PROMISE)

We have tried to create a common-sense program in this book that gives you every advantage in your quest to quit smoking. This approach is one that anyone can follow to achieve success. You have read the latest medical and scientific information on how to quit, so that facts and expertise could add to your motivation. Remember that there is no magic method. To quit smoking is an arduous yet achievable goal. Like any worthwhile endeavor, effort is required. In the end, only you have the ability to free yourself from cigarettes. With preparation, knowledge, and motivation, you can and will succeed—no if's, and's, or butts!

Good Luck!

Appendix

There are a number of national organizations that can be valuable resources to you. Here are just a few of the best-known organizations, with addresses and telephone numbers for each of them.

American Cancer Society
1599 Clifton Road, N.E.
Atlanta, GA 32329
404-320-3333

American Cancer Society
19 West 56th Street
New York, NY 10019
212-586-8700

American Heart Association
7272 Greenville Avenue
Dallas, TX 75231
214-373-6300

American Lung Association
1740 Broadway
New York, NY 10019
212-315-8700

National Cancer Institute
National Institutes of Health
Building 31, Room 10A24
Bethesda, MD 20892
800-4-CANCER, or
800-422-6237

Office on Smoking and Health
U.S. Department of Health
  Services
5600 Fishers Lane
Park Building, Room 110
Rockville, MD 20857
301-443-1575

Index